FIFTY PLACES TO RUN

BEFORE YOU DIE

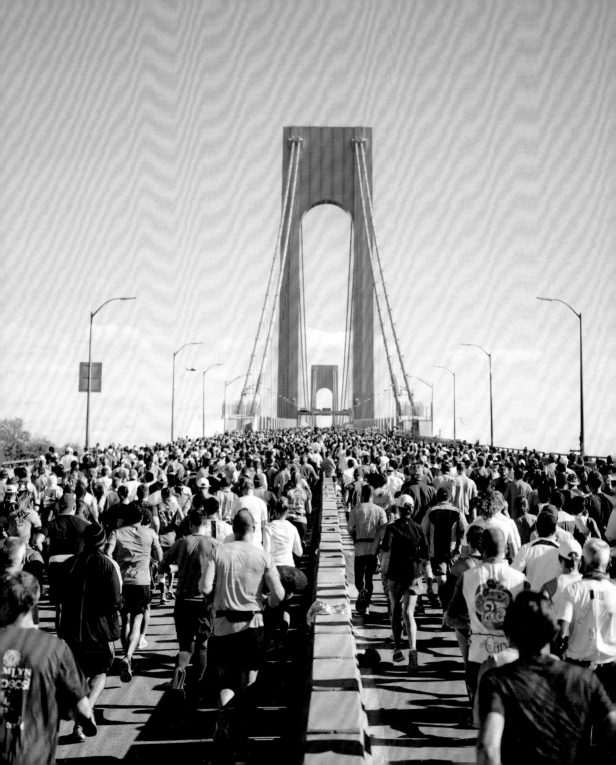

FIFTY PLACES TO
RUN
BEFORE YOU DIE

Running Experts Share
the World's Greatest Destinations

Chris Santella

FOREWORD BY THOM GILLIGAN

ABRAMS IMAGE
NEW YORK

This book is for my girls, Cassidy, Annabel, and Deidre,
and for everyone who's ever laced up their sneakers to hit the asphalt or trail.

Fifty Places to Drink Beer Before You Die

Fifty Places to Camp Before You Die

Fifty Places to Paddle Before You Die

Fifty Places to Bike Before You Die

Fifty Places to Fly Fish Before You Die

Fifty More Places to Fly Fish Before You Die

Fifty Places to Ski & Snowboard Before You Die

Fifty Places to Sail Before You Die

Fifty Places to Go Birding Before You Die

Fifty Places to Dive Before You Die

Fifty Places to Hike Before You Die

Fifty Places to Play Golf Before You Die

Fifty More Places to Play Golf Before You Die

Once in a Lifetime Trips

Fifty Favorite Fly-Fishing Tales

Why I Fly Fish

The Hatch Is On!

The Tug Is the Drug

CAT WARS (with Dr. Peter Marra)

Contents

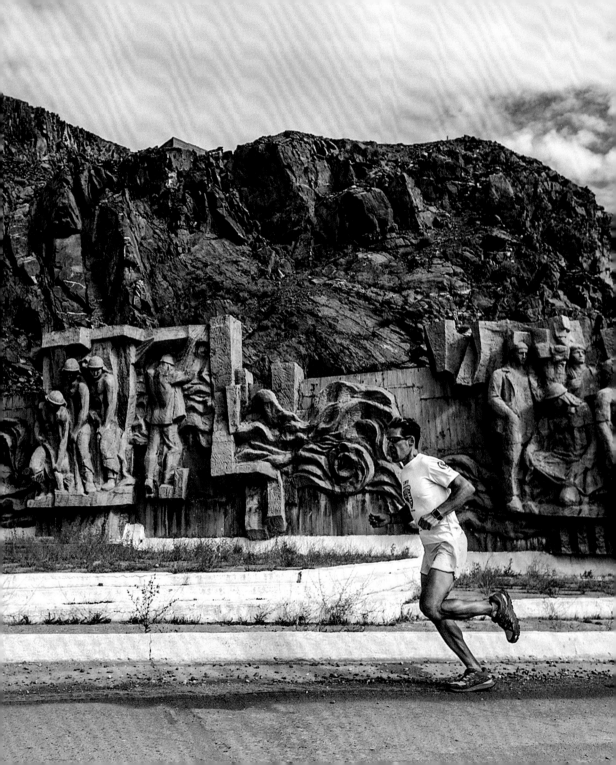

ACKNOWLEDGMENTS

This book would not have been possible without the generous assistance of the runners—marathoners and trail runners, ultra-runners and harriers—who shared their time and experience to help bring these fifty great running venues to life. To these men and women, I offer the most heartfelt thanks. I also wish to extend thanks to Mark Weinstein at Rodale, who made several important introductions on my behalf . . . and to my former editor, Jennifer Levesque, for introducing me to Mark! I want to acknowledge the fine efforts of my agent, Stephanie Kip Rostan; my editors, Samantha Weiner, Ashley Albert, and David Blatty; designer Anna Christian; and copy editor Anna Dobbin, who all helped bring the book into being.

A special thanks goes out to Dr. Ware Kuschner, who is one of the most dedicated runners I know and a constant inspiration. Finally, I want to express my gratitude to my wife, Deidre, and my daughters, Cassidy and Annabel, for their patience with my peripatetic lifestyle . . . and to my mother, Tina, and recently departed father, Andy, who always encouraged me to pursue my passions.

OPPOSITE:
Dean Karnazes passes a Soviet relief mural in Talas, Kyrgyzstan, as part of his Silk Road sports diplomacy run in 2016.

FOREWORD

Fifty Places to Run Before You Die has enough gems to keep every runner's bags packed and passport handy for a lifetime. Featuring running events on all seven continents, this book will help dedicated runners compile a manageable bucket list—for every taste and budget.

Are you looking to run one of the Abbott World Marathon Majors? Check out the chapters on Boston, Chicago, London, Berlin, or New York. Or perhaps you prefer a classic 10K, such as the Peachtree Road Race in Atlanta. How about San Francisco's riotous Bay to Breakers? If you have a more adventurous spirit, check out the Conquer the Wall Marathon in China, the Madagascar Marathon, or the Amazing Maasai Marathon in Kenya. Each event promises to be a memorable or even life-changing experience.

Travel is an integral part of the runner's lifestyle. I have met many runners who no longer consider "fun-in-the-sun" vacations. As type-A personalities, they have upgraded their activity levels to "run-for-fun" vacations. Some running events even cater to the whole family with simultaneously held races of varying distances. This tome is also perfect for any running club looking to plan a road trip or an overseas adventure.

Whether your goal is to race in every state—or every continent—*Fifty Places to Run Before You Die* will not only help you find unforgettable runs in major cities, remote villages, and exotic landscapes; it will help you break through the touristic veneer for an elbow-to-elbow experience with local runners. There is no better way to explore the world than one stride at a time.

Where is your next running destination?

—THOM GILLIGAN, CEO AND FOUNDER, MARATHON TOURS & TRAVEL

INTRODUCTION

At various points in my life, I've tried to take up running . . . but with a bad back, poor wind, and a few too many pounds, it's never quite taken. Yet I've always been impressed by friends who adhere to a regular running schedule. It's so simple, so primal. And by the looks of them, so healthy! I've also been intrigued watching some of these friends "train up" for a special challenge, be it a 10K, a marathon, or something even more ambitious. Do people really run a hundred miles over mountain ranges without sleep—and do it in less than twenty-four hours?!

I wrote *Fifty Places to Run Before You Die* for those who appreciate the challenges running affords . . . and for the opportunity to share these experiences with fellow runners while seeing a bit of the world.

"What makes a destination or event a place to run before you die?" you might ask. Is it the chance to run in the footsteps of champion athletes who have come before you? To explore an unfamiliar city or country from the unique vantage points offered by sweeping boulevards or mountain trails? To immerse yourself in the beauty of stunning natural settings while pushing past physical boundaries? Or is it simply the opportunity to surround yourself with thousands—or tens of thousands—of like-minded people? The answer is all of the above, and more. One thing I knew when I began this project: I was *not* the person to assemble this list. So I followed a recipe that served me well in my thirteen previous Fifty Places books—I sought the advice of dedicated professionals. To write *Fifty Places to Run Before You Die*, I interviewed a host of people from the running world and asked them to share some of their favorite experiences. These experts range from celebrated Olympic athletes (including Steve Moneghetti and David Bedford) to endurance running legends (Dean Karnazes, Tim Twietmeyer, and newcomer Jim Walmsley) to travel authorities (Thom Gilligan, Karen Hoch, and Bart Yasso) . . . and even a public radio star (Peter Sagal). Some spoke of venues that are near and dear to their hearts, places where they've built their professional reputations; others spoke of places they've visited only once but that made a profound impression. There is no shortage of ways to feel a connection with a place—or a sport for that matter—as evidenced in these pages. (To give a sense of the breadth of the interviewees' backgrounds, a bio of each individual is included after each essay.)

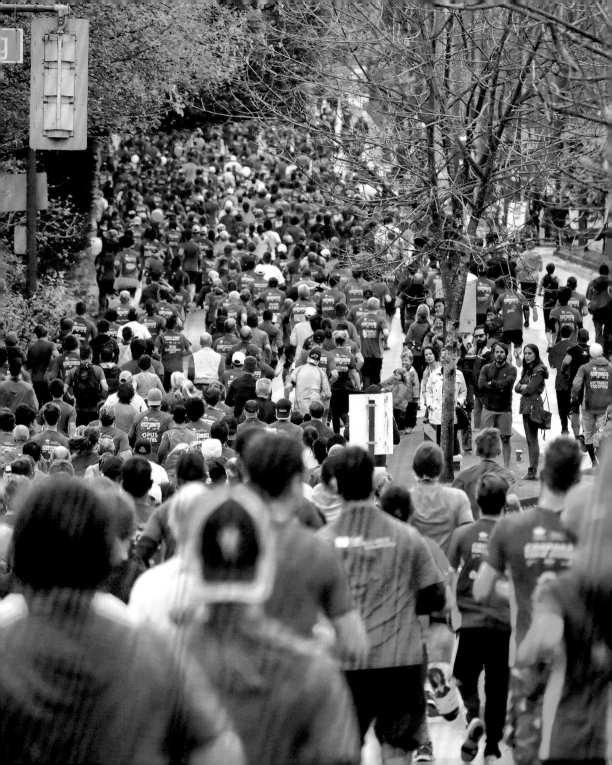

For some people, running is a low-pressure 10K with a great party afterward; for others, it may not begin to count as running until you've logged at least thirty or forty miles. *Fifty Places to Run Before You Die* attempts to capture the full spectrum of running experiences—on road, off-road, 10K, marathon, endurance . . . and some runs that defy easy classification. While the book describes fifty great venues, it does not attempt to rank the quality of the experiences afforded by each place. Such ranking would, of course, be largely subjective.

To help readers actualize their running aspirations, I have provided brief "If You Go" information at the end of each chapter, which includes registration details for formal events. The "If You Go" information is by no means comprehensive but should give would-be travelers a starting point for planning their trip.

One of the beauties of running is that just about anywhere you might find yourself, you can lace up your sneakers, step outside your door, and reap the benefits of a good run. Yet a trip to a storied event or dream venue can create memories for a lifetime. It's my hope that this little book will inspire you to embark on some new running adventures of your own.

I may even try to take it up again myself!

OPPOSITE: *The Vancouver Sun Run takes runners through the heart of one of North America's most beautiful cities.*

NEXT PAGE: *Europe's tallest mountain, Mont Blanc, looms over contestants throughout the grueling Ultra-Trail du Mont-Blanc (UTMB).*

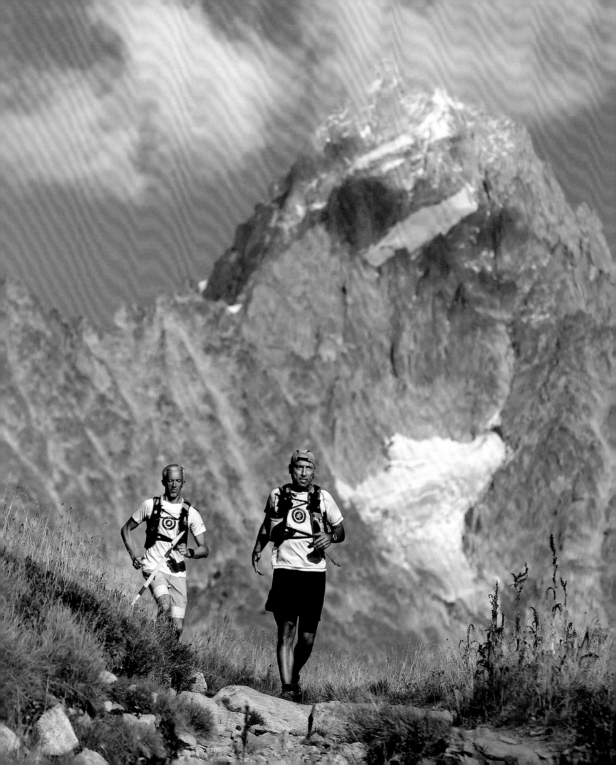

The Destinations

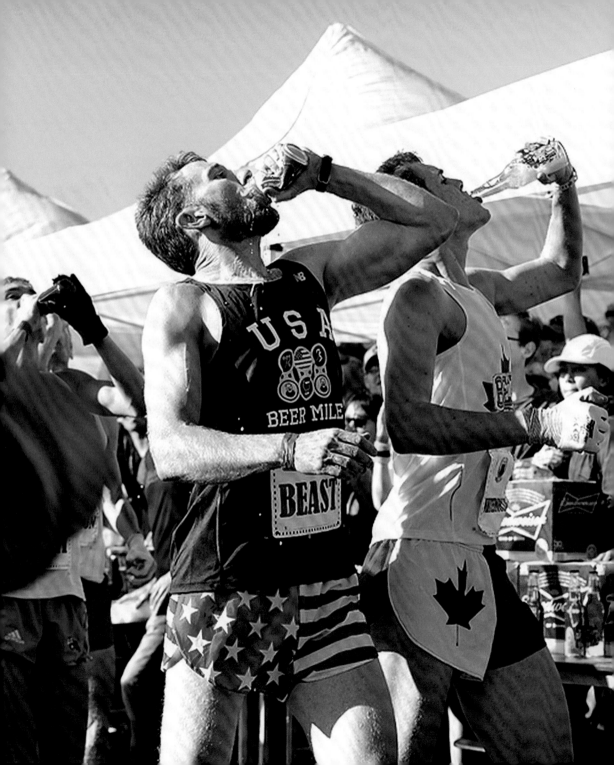

BEER MILE WORLD CLASSIC

RECOMMENDED BY **Corey Bellemore**

It's not uncommon for runners to enjoy a convivial beer at the conclusion of an event while recounting the day. It is a somewhat more finite group who imbibe beer—forty-eight ounces, to be precise—while running competitively. These are the beer milers.

"I came into the beer mile like most people do," Corey Bellemore began. "At the end of our university season, we usually do a beer mile as a team, just for fun. After trying it out, I knew I was pretty decent at it and could run much faster if I actually went for it. [In the summer of 2016], after an eleven-hour workday, a friend came over with a six-pack of beer and wanted me to head to the track by my house to attempt the world record. We agreed to tape it, but if it went poorly no one would ever know about it. It ended up going well, and I beat the 'world record' by eight seconds, with a time of four minutes, thirty-nine seconds. We posted the video online and it went viral, with articles being written about it immediately. The next morning I woke up to many messages, including one from a Facebook account called the Beer Mile World Classic, which was a big beer mile race going on that weekend in London. They offered to fly me out that night so I could participate in the race."

While there's some suggestion that runners experimented with variations of the beer mile concept in the early 1980s, *Runner's World* traces its genesis to a track in Burlington, Ontario, on an August night in 1989. Seven young running friends (including Graham Hood, who would later run the 1,500 meters in the Olympics) had concocted a plan—drink four beers, sprint four laps, beer, lap, beer, lap, etc. (As this was Ontario, the beer was likely Molson or Labatt.) Each runner lined up four unopened cans of beer for himself at the starting line, the timer was started, and the race began. The runners guessed that the beer would pose challenges, but those challenges were not what they'd expected;

*OPPOSITE:
A scene from
the first annual
Beer Mile
World Classic
at Treasure
Island in San
Francisco in
2015. Lewis Kent
(the Canadian
runner) won the
event that year.*

the alcohol wasn't a problem as much as the carbonation, which creates a tangible level of discomfort. Happy with their experiment, some of the original runners carried the contest along with them to Queen's University in Kingston, Ontario. T-shirts were made. And the beer mile became a small part of the running canon.

"The beer mile was once an underground thing with no real media attention," Corey continued, "but that changed once Lewis Kent broke the world record in 2016, and our agent Kris Mychasiw began to elevate the sport. It's an untapped market that the average person is very interested in."

As the beer mile has come out of the shadows, a codified set of rules has emerged:

1. Each competitor drinks four cans of beer and runs four laps, ideally on a track (start—beer, then lap, then beer, then lap, then beer, then lap, then beer, then lap—finish).

2. Beer must be consumed before the lap is begun, within the transition area, which is the ten-meter zone before the start/finish line on a four-hundred-meter track.

3. The race begins with the drinking of the first beer in the last meter of the transition zone to ensure the competitors run a complete mile (1,609 meters).

4. Women also drink four beers in four laps.

5. Competitors must drink canned beer, and the cans should not be less than 355 milliliters (the standard can volume) or twelve ounces (the imperial equivalent). Bottles may be substituted for cans as long as they are at least twelve ounces (355 milliliters) in volume.

6. No specialized cans or bottles that give an advantage by allowing the beer to pour at a faster rate may be used.

7. Beer cans must not be tampered with in any manner. Puncturing the can, apart from opening it by the tab at the top, is not permitted; this prevents shotgunning. The same applies to bottles—no straws or other aids that would increase the speed of pouring are allowed.

8. Beer must be a minimum of 5 percent alcohol by volume. Hard ciders and lemonades will not suffice. The beer must be a fermented alcoholic beverage brewed from malted cereal grains and flavored with hops.

9. Each beer can must not be opened until the competitor enters the transition zone on each lap.

10. Competitors who *evacuate* any beer before they finish the race must complete one penalty lap at the end of the race (immediately after the completion of their fourth lap). Note: Vomiting more than once during the race requires only one penalty lap at the end.

Corey ended up flying to London and running in the Beer Mile World Classic at Allianz Park. "It was my first time running in a competitive and electronically timed beer mile," he recalled. "It was the most spontaneous trip I've ever taken in my life. I got in late Saturday morning and then competed Sunday morning, where I broke my own world record, running a time of four minutes, thirty-four seconds."

The Beer Mile World Classic shifts locales each year. As of this writing, it's been held in San Francisco and London, and it is likely to be held in Copenhagen in 2018.

When asked to share a few beer mile secrets, Corey offered four tips:

1. Get in the best mile shape you can.

2. Find a chugging method that enables you to drink as fast as the beer comes out of the bottle.

3. Learn to run comfortably with a full stomach or a stomach full of fluids.

4. Find a beer that works best for you. For me, that's a pilsner called Mythology from Flying Monkeys Brewery.

How does one celebrate a successful beer mile? More beer, naturally! "At the beer mile events I've gone to, you usually see many familiar faces," Corey shared. "It's fun to catch up with those guys and live it up for the night with them."

COREY BELLEMORE is currently the world beer mile champion and record holder and an accomplished track and field athlete without a beer in hand. As a student at the University of Windsor, he won the eight hundred meters at the Canadian National Championships in 2015 and was named one of the university's athletes of the year in 2016. Corey is sponsored by Adidas Running, Flying Monkeys Brewery, Run Gum, and Infinit Nutrition Canada.

If You Go

▶ **Getting There:** The venue for the Beer Mile World Classic shifts each year.

▶ **Best Time to Visit:** The event is held in mid-summer.

▶ **Race Information:** Learn more about the Beer Mile World Classic at beermileworld classic.com. Details about other beer mile events can be found at beermile.com.

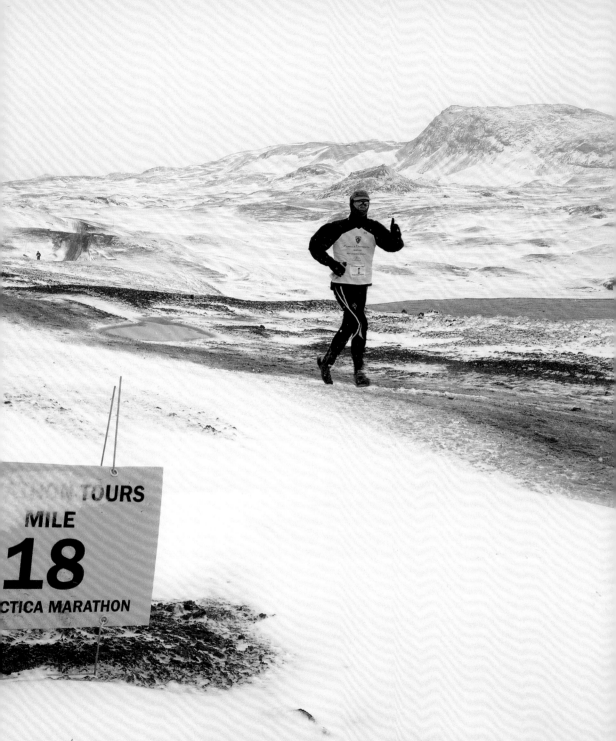

ANTARCTICA MARATHON

RECOMMENDED BY **Bart Yasso**

In recent years, Antarctica has seen a considerable increase in the number of human visitors during the brief austral summer. Many people come on large cruise ships that must maintain a comfortable distance from terra firma. A lesser number of visitors travel on smaller vessels that can be maneuvered closer to the seventh continent's ice and rocks.

And a few hundred visitors each year not only touch down on the landmass, but run there, competing in the world's southernmost marathon.

"When Thom Gilligan from Marathon Tours & Travel reached out to me about running in Antarctica, my interest was piqued," Bart Yasso recalled. "I saw it as an opportunity to get to the last continent. It seemed like a once-in-a-lifetime trip."

Antarctica is not one of the world's most welcoming places. This is evidenced by the fact that there are no indigenous people on the continent, even though Antarctica encompasses more than five million square miles, roughly 1.5 times the size of the United States! A great majority of the landmass—an estimated 98 percent—consists of ice and snow that has an average thickness of seven thousand feet; scientists believe that up to 70 percent of the world's fresh water is contained here.) During the winter months, when temperatures hover in the balmy range of -40 to -90 degrees, seawater surrounding the continent freezes up to two hundred miles offshore, covering an area even larger than Antarctica's landmass. In the summer (December through March), the freeze recedes, and a brief window opens for sailing to the more northerly portions of Antarctica.

The first Antarctica Marathon was run in 1995. Thom Gilligan chose the location, King George Island—just north of the Antarctic Peninsula and technically part of the South Shetland Islands—for two reasons. First, there were rough gravel roads connecting four of the scientific bases on the island (those operated by Uruguay, Russia, Chile, and

OPPOSITE:
The Antarctica Marathon and Half Marathon is the world's southernmost running race.

21

China) that would facilitate marking out a course and minimize impact on this ecologically sensitive land; second, the existing infrastructure would expedite access should a medical emergency arise. The course runs first to the Uruguayan base and back, and then through the Russian, Chilean, and Chinese bases. To reach 26.2 miles, runners loop this course four times over terrain that's a mix of rocks, mud, and glacier. "Some people got fancy in terms of footwear with spikes in their shoes," Bart continued, "though I didn't think they were necessary. The mud that emerged when the snow would melt in the sun was the hardest part to deal with. There's no shoe designed for that."

Some have joked that the real marathon involved in running the Antarctica Marathon is getting there. Suffice it to say, one doesn't merely jet in, run, and jet out. Runners first fly into Buenos Aires, where they have a few days to explore the "Paris of South America." From here, you'll fly to Ushuaia in Tierra del Fuego, the world's southernmost city. Next you'll board one of two ships for the roughly two-day crossing of the Drake Passage— almost five hundred miles, from Cape Horn to the Shetland Islands at the northern tip of the continent. As you push farther south, you'll pass through alleys of icebergs— cracking, rolling, with massive chunks calving off—and the wildness of the seventh continent will begin to unfold. Upon reaching King George, race organizers will go ashore to set up the course; runners will have the chance to board Zodiac rafts and do some nature watching. You're sure to encounter massive rookeries of penguins and colonies of seals, along with the pods of humpback whales that migrate here to feed on krill. The following day, the race is run; after another few days of exploring, you'll cross the Drake Passage again en route to Ushuaia, Buenos Aires, and home.

Despite these time-commitment and logistical challenges, the two hundred spots reserved each year for the Antarctica Marathon and Half Marathon are booked several years in advance.

"There wasn't much wildlife on the course," Bart recalled, "with the exception of birds called skuas. They were nesting along the course, and as we'd run, some would dive-bomb us. They'd lock eyes with you and fly right at your head. As I'd duck, they'd slap me in the back of the head with their webbed feet. They wouldn't attack larger packs of runners, but you didn't want to be one of the front or back runners. I have to say, I'd face down a bear before one of these birds." A more amiable animal encounter came after the race. "I remember being in a Zodiac and there were minke whales coming up next to us. They weren't aggressive, but they were still intimidating, as they were twice as wide and twice as long as the raft. Still, you could feel the peacefulness of their presence."

BART YASSO is the chief running officer for *Runner's World*. He joined the magazine in 1987 to develop the groundbreaking *Runner's World* Race Sponsorship program, creating a vehicle for the magazine to work with more than seven thousand races representing four million runners per year. Inducted into the Running USA Hall of Champions, Bart also invented the Yasso 800s, a marathon-training schedule used by thousands around the world. He is one of the few people to have completed races on all seven continents, from the Antarctica Half Marathon to the Mount Kilimanjaro Marathon. In 1987, he won the US National Biathlon Long Course Championship and won the Smoky Mountain Marathon in 1998. He has also completed the Ironman five times and the Badwater 135® through Death Valley. Bart has cycled, unsupported and by himself, across the United States twice.

If You Go

▶ **Getting There:** To participate in an Antarctic running event, you'll need to sign on with a booking agent like Marathon Tours & Travel (marathontours.com). Most groups collect in Buenos Aires (which is served by most major carriers). From there, runners fly to Ushuaia and join a boat to sail south.

▶ **Best Time to Visit:** The Antarctica Marathon and Half Marathon is held in mid-March.

▶ **Race Information:** The event described above is orchestrated by Marathon Tours & Travel (617-242-7845; marathontours.com). All transportation (from Buenos Aires) and accommodations are included.

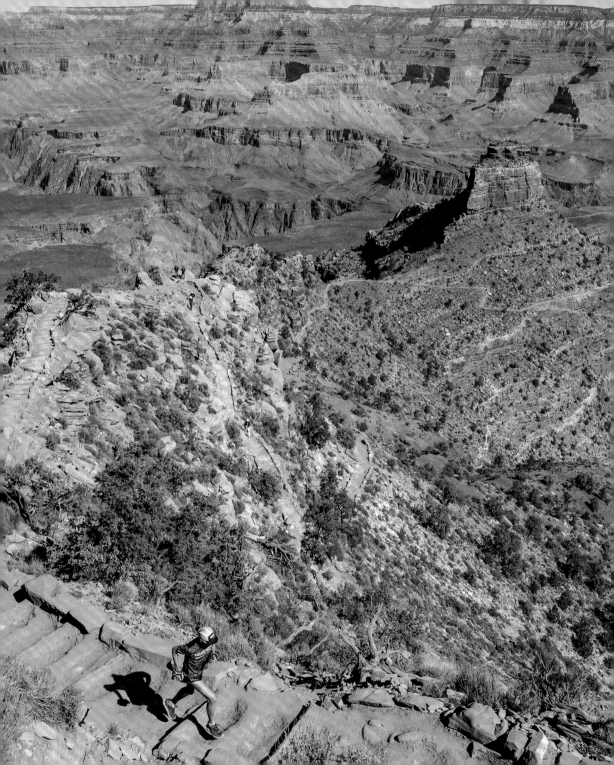

GRAND CANYON

RECOMMENDED BY **Jim Walmsley**

Neither the deepest nor widest gorge in the world, the Grand Canyon is nonetheless recognized as one of the planet's most awe-inspiring erosion events—a 277-mile-long chasm that yawns from four to eighteen miles wide and reaches depths of more than a mile, a seemingly endless series of abrupt cliffs and gentle slopes. Millions of visitors will peer down into the canyon in wonder from the South or North Rim. Tens of thousands will hike into the canyon, perhaps going as far as Phantom Ranch. Some of those will complete the Trans-Canyon (or Rim to Rim hike). Even fewer people will run that distance in one fell swoop, gaining and losing approximately twelve thousand feet in elevation. Fewer still will complete the Rim to Rim to Rim run, a feat that's high on many trail runners' bucket lists.

Jim Walmsley took things one step further in October of 2016; he set out to best the Fastest Known Time (FKT) on the "R2R2R," a record of six hours, twenty-one minutes, forty-seven seconds that had been set by Rob Krar. "Rob established this FKT as one of the hardest, most competitive FKTs in the world," Jim said. "I have nothing but the utmost respect for what Rob has been able to do in ultra-running. He is a big reason why this record is such a big target for many people and why many people don't even want to attempt it."

The route that a majority of runners will take in their attempts to tackle the R2R2R begins at the South Kaibab Trailhead on the Grand Canyon's South Rim. This route descends into the canyon to Phantom Ranch, passes through a series of box canyons en route to Cottonwood Campground, and then ascends to the North Kaibab Trailhead. This route is forty-two miles in length, and much of the trail is well maintained. While the mileage may not be of great concern to the seasoned ultra-runner, the extreme elevation

OPPOSITE:
Running across
the Grand
Canyon is a
tremendous
challenge;
running back
and forth in
less than six
hours seems
beyond human
capability.

gains and losses—between 10,500 and 12,000 feet down and the same back up, depend-ing on whom you talk to—are sobering. At times, the grade is 60 percent.

Any effort to run back and forth across the Grand Canyon requires considerable training and preparation. One of Jim's key concerns going into his record attempt was the timing of his start. "I planned my start time for around four thirty A.M.," he continued, "because if I could make it to the North Rim by seven thirty A.M., I would be guaranteed to not hit a mule train for the first thirty-five miles." To navigate a trail that can be challenging for walkers in full daylight, Jim outfitted himself with two head lamps—one upside-down around his waist, one around his forehead. (The former would enable him to better see the shadows of bumps and rocks.) From a running perspective, he knew that steep descents could pose a challenge. "Anyone who has ever run in the canyon has learned one thing," Jim added. "You go down too fast, you blow your legs and you can't climb back out. I have learned to withstand bombing down the canyon while keeping lots of power to climb back out South Kaibab in under seventy minutes."

There are many impasses standing between a runner and a successful R2R2R, let alone a record-breaking attempt. One that Jim didn't anticipate was a mountain lion. "I was in the narrow box canyons just a couple miles past Phantom Ranch," he described. "Huge cliff walls were on my left, the Bright Angel Creek on my left as well, and another huge cliff wall was on my right. Fifty yards in front of me, I saw some really bright, white reflections. There aren't many, if any, fluorescent markings on the trail, so that got ruled out pretty quickly. I soon realized these weren't like any deer eyes I'd ever seen before. This was something else, and it was something big. I started shouting at it at the top of my lungs and making loud noises. Meanwhile, I was running full speed at it. I don't think I even took into consideration that the mountain lion didn't have anywhere to go. All six feet and 140 pounds of me, warrior-shouting at it, was enough to trigger one of the most athletic things I've ever seen in my life. The animal turned to its left and made an enor-mous leap up the cliff wall. The next mile or so, I was flying."

By the time Jim reached the North Rim kiosk, 2:46:08 had elapsed—some five minutes faster than the current FKT for an R2R. There were a few moments when he considered calling it good, but such considerations were short-lived. It wasn't long before he was dashing past Cottonwood Campground, pausing at Phantom Ranch for some water and a potty stop, and finding himself with the final six-odd miles—and 5,200-foot elevation gain—of South Kaibab to conquer. "It was a really hard grind the last few miles up South Kaibab," he recalled. "I felt I was prepared for the mental challenge. I had hoped I could hold up better physically. Luckily, I wanted it bad enough. Once you crest Cedar Ridge, it's not long before someone with a good eye might be able to spot a runner from the top of the trailhead. I kept this in mind, as I knew my parents and my friends were anxiously waiting for this moment. I mustered what felt like a decent jog from Cedar Ridge. I knew I had the first ever sub-six-hour R2R2R in the bag at this point. I kept following the sounds of the cheering from above. The end was here. I walked in the last few steps to the kiosk at the South Kaibab Trailhead and slammed my hand down on it like a contestant from *American Ninja Warrior*. I finally got to collapse on the bench that's around the kiosk. That. Hurt. A lot!"

Jim's FKT, incidentally, was logged at five hours, fifty-five minutes, and twenty seconds.

JIM WALMSLEY is a HOKA ONE ONE–sponsored ultra-runner based in Flagstaff, Arizona. A former NCAA standout at the United States Air Force Academy, Jim took the trail ultra world by storm in 2016 with a series of wins and course records at competitive races. His aggressive racing style, even over ultra-distances, gained him acclaim, as did his speed record in the Grand Canyon's R2R2R route, where he was the first person ever to break six hours.

If You Go

▶ **Getting There:** Most R2R2R runners will begin at the South Rim. The nearest airports are in Phoenix (served by most carriers) and Flagstaff, which is served by Alaska Airlines (800-252-7522; alaskaair.com) and US Airways (800-428-4322; usairways.com).

▶ **Best Time to Visit:** March/April or October/November, as temperatures are cooler and there's less traffic on the trails.

▶ **Running Information:** A number of websites, including Runner's World (runnersworld.com) and Competitor (running.competitor.com), provide helpful tips (including training regimens) for preparing to tackle the R2R2R.

▶ **Accommodations:** Xanterra South Rim (888-29-PARKS; grandcanyonlodges.com) offers a number of accommodation options around the South Rim.

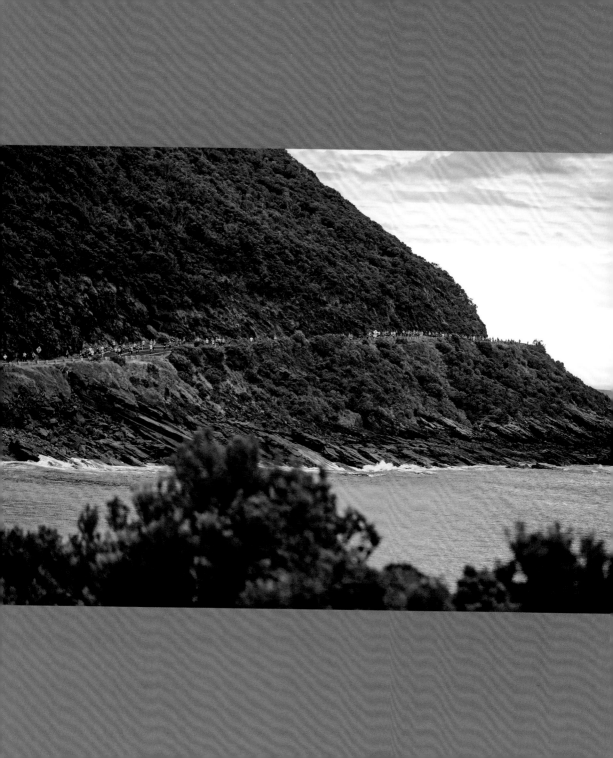

GREAT OCEAN ROAD MARATHON

RECOMMENDED BY **Steve Moneghetti**

If Australia has an iconic stretch of highway, it would have to be the Great Ocean Road. The road spans 150 miles in the state of Victoria, hugging the coast from Torquay in the east to Allansford in the west. It passes through several national parks and is bordered by the Pacific. A favorite section of the road is near the village of Port Campbell, where the ocean is dotted with awe-inspiring limestone formations, most notably the Twelve Apostles, the Grotto, and the London Arch. Back in 2005, Steve Moneghetti was part of a team that set out to create a race that would honor this august piece of macadam.

"The Great Ocean Road is for Australians what the section of Highway 1 in California that stretches along Big Sur is for Americans," Steve began. "Tourists come from far and wide to travel the road. May is the shoulder season before our winter, and most of the people who come to the coast of Victoria for holiday are gone at this time. Some of the hotel owners down there were hoping to get a running event going to stir up some tourism activity. I went down to Apollo Bay, a town along the road, to meet with these folks, who were very enthusiastic. On my way home, my wife called. I told her that there were a bunch of blokes down here who thought they were going to get the authorities to close down the road for a race. It would never happen. One of the guys called a few days later with good news—the authorities were going to let the race happen."

The course that Steve and his mates devised begins at the town of Lorne and moves west to its finish line at Apollo Bay. "I call it a pub crawl," he continued, "as it starts in front of a pub and concludes in front of another. When you drive the Great Ocean Road, you can't focus on the scenery too much, as it's a fairly dangerous road if you're not paying attention. When you're running it, you can absorb the environment you're in." (In addition to the marathon, there's an ultra event [sixty kilometers], a half marathon, a 14K, a 6K, and a 1.5K.)

OPPOSITE:
The Great Ocean
Road has few
level stretches
but consistently
spectacular views.

The Great Ocean Road is not the sort of course where one can expect to set a personal best. "The road undulates most of the way," Steve continued, "and that makes it quite challenging. There are no flat sections to speak of. You're often going up a bluff, then ducking down into an inlet, past a coastal village, then up another bluff. When you're on a bluff, you can often look across and see where you'll be in ten minutes' time. It may seem close, but distances can be deceiving. At one point, about twenty-five kilometers into the race, you reach a spot called Cape Patton. Here, you come out of a coastal village, head up a fairly steep climb where you're protected, and come out on a bluff where you're open to the wind. It will stand you upright. This is the highest point on the course. From here, you can look southwest across the water and hills and see the Apollo Bay lighthouse. You still have twenty kilometers to get there, but this sneak peek offers encouragement." Not far from Cape Patton there's a heavily forested bend called Koala Corner that's often frequented by one of Australia's totemic mammals. "There's no guarantee you'll see them, of course," Steve added, "but they are often present."

There are several points of entry to the Great Ocean Road Marathon. Some will over-night in Lorne, the starting point. Others will stay in Apollo Bay, the ending point. For those runners, there's the singular experience of driving the route in reverse before the run. "There's a great camaraderie on the bus," Steve described. "You may be seated next to someone you've never met, but you're about to share something special. As you ride up and down the hills, you're thinking, 'How am I going to get over this?' It adds to the anticipation." The race's conclusion is equally exceptional. "I've finished a lot of events around the world, but there's something special about the conclusion at Apollo Bay. It seems that everyone from the community lines the road for four hundred meters. Even though the road closure impacts the community's life, they've really embraced it. Everyone is made to feel like such a winner, even if you're a seven-hour runner." A host of coffee shops, pubs, and eateries await at the finish line to satisfy your well-earned cravings. The Pacific also awaits you. "The water is pretty chilly in May," Steve added, "but a number of runners will wade in together and share their war stories."

Like at Big Sur, the weather along the Great Ocean Road can be changeable, and fog is not an infrequent visitor. Steve recalled a Sunday morning in May when the race was still in its infancy. "It was the second year, and I woke up in Lorne, quite early. I went to the starting line, and people were already assembling. The weather had closed in, thick gray clouds, and I felt like it was going to be a hard day—and would a hard day this early in the marathon's history impact its future success? As we were standing at the starting line, preparing to run, the clouds just cleared away, and the sun started rising—a huge red sun across the horizon. I couldn't help but think that the marathon gods were smiling on us. I realized that the Great Ocean Road Marathon was going to have legs and a future."

STEVE MONEGHETTI has represented Australia in the men's marathon at four Commonwealth Games, winning gold (1994), silver (1990), and two bronze (1986 and 1998) medals. He achieved three top-ten finishes in his four appearances at the Olympic Games (1988, 1992, 1996, and 2000) and attended six IAAF World Championships, winning a bronze medal in the marathon event in Athens in 1997. Steve retired as an athlete in 2000. He served as mayor of the Commonwealth Games Village at the Melbourne 2006 Commonwealth Games and as the Australian team's chef de mission for the Delhi 2010 Commonwealth Games. From 2001 to 2010, Steve served as chair of the Victorian Institute of Sport and also chaired the Victorian State Review into Physical and Sport Education in Schools. Steve received an Australian Sports Medal in 2000 and a Centenary Medal in 2001. In 2014 he was awarded an Order of Australia medal for significant service to athletics as a marathon runner, administrator, and mentor to young athletes, and he was named director at the Australian Sports Commission in 2015.

If You Go

▶ **Getting There:** Lorne is roughly two hours from Melbourne, which is served by many major carriers from Los Angeles, including United (800-864-8331; united.com), Qantas (800-227-4500; qantas.com), and American (800-433-7300; aa.com).

▶ **Best Time to Visit:** The Great Ocean Road Marathon (and the other Great Ocean Road events) is held the third weekend in May.

▶ **Race Information:** Registration information and other race details reside at the Great Ocean Road Running Festival website (greatoceanroadrunfest.com.au).

▶ **Accommodations:** Lodging options in Apollo Bay are available from the Apollo Bay Visitor Information Centre (+61 13689297; visitgreatoceanroad.org.au); options in Lorne are available from the Lorne Visitor Information Centre (+61 13891152).

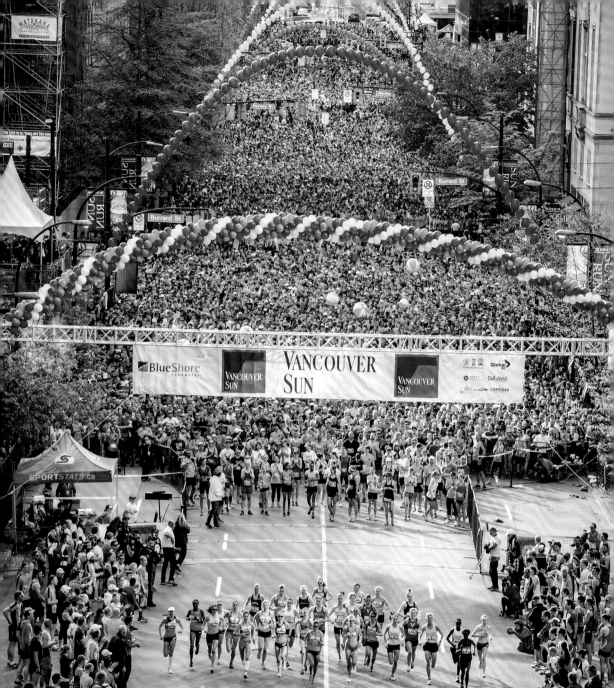

VANCOUVER SUN RUN

RECOMMENDED BY **Gord Fisher**

Vancouver, the stunning seaside city at the southwest corner of British Columbia, has a reputation for a health-conscious and outdoors-oriented citizenry. It's the kind of place where people don't *watch* things; they *do* things. Given its proximity to wonderful natural amenities, it's pretty easy to enjoy the outdoors.

But back in the early 1980s, a few Vancouverites thought they could do a little better.

"It was 1984, and at the time I was assistant managing editor of the *Vancouver Sun* [the largest newspaper in Vancouver]," Gord Fisher recalled. "Three former Olympians—Ken Elmer, Dr. Doug [Clement], and Diane Clement—along with Dr. Jack Taunton, who's known as British Columbia's 'father of running,' came to the paper with the idea of a run. Their objectives were centered on raising the profile and funding of local elite runners, with a focus on health and community, all to be celebrated under the umbrella of a 10K event. They went to the *Sun*'s publisher first, who was only lukewarm to the idea. He didn't see the connection quite the way they did; however, their efforts were supported by leaders in the newsroom, who embraced the idea, sensing that it was something they could do a lot with. And the publisher eventually agreed.

"I still remember that first run in 1985 very well. We had 3,500 participants. At the time, we thought it was a phenomenal turnout. We were in awe of its success. A few years back, the participation level hit fifty thousand." (The Sun Run is now the second-largest timed 10K in the world.)

To this day, the Vancouver Sun Run subscribes to its initial mission: to be Canada's leading and most influential 10K race inspiring healthy, active lifestyles for people of all ages and fitness levels. (The likelihood of seeing the sun as you run in Vancouver in late April is fairly low; weather statistics suggest 90 percent cloudiness for April.)

OPPOSITE:
Waves of runners depart at the Vancouver Sun Run— the second-largest timed 10K in the world.

It would be difficult to create a more compelling setting for an urban 10K race. Vancouver's city center is bordered by water on three sides—Burrard Inlet to the north, False Creek to the south, and English Bay to the west. On its northern tip is Stanley Park, one of North America's largest urban green spaces. The North Shore Mountains are in view on all but the foggiest days, further enhancing the city's natural beauty. Vancouver's diverse and cosmopolitan community (including Canada's largest Chinatown) now attracts nearly ten million tourists a year. (Vancouver's élan was not harmed by its hosting of the 2010 Winter Olympics and Paralympics.) Most who come from outside of the province to participate in the Sun Run extend their stay to enjoy the city's vibrant cultural and food scene.

Given Vancouver's beauty, it wasn't difficult to map out a visually stunning course. The Sun Run begins on Georgia Street near the center of the downtown area and then heads north to Stanley Park. Here, it reverses direction, heading south along the West End (looking out over English Bay) before crossing the Burrard Street Bridge. From here it heads east along False Creek before crossing the water once again on the Cambie Street Bridge. The race finishes in front of BC Place Stadium, home of the BC Lions (Canadian football) and the Vancouver Whitecaps (Major League Soccer). "There's really not a bad stretch of the run," Gord continued, "though there are a few parts that stand out. It's hard to beat the start, almost fifty thousand people, all geared up and ready to go under waving banners with bands playing. Watching the runners set off in waves is a compelling sight, whether you're looking down from a nearby deck or are in the middle of the action. I also love the approach coming into Stanley Park Lost Lagoon [a pond in the park]. It's so beautiful, you want to stop and look around—many do. When you get to the Burrard Street Bridge, there's usually a sea of people, but the crowds are not a bother, as you're crossing a scenic piece of water with mountains in the background. The course is generally flat, but this is one spot that's a bit of a test. The same can be said of the Cambie Street Bridge, but at this point, you're nearly done. There's a tremendous sense of community as runners enter the stadium. People from all different walks of life are brought together." True to its mission, the Sun Run attracts a wide swath of the running community—from serious amateur runners and wheelchair athletes to casual walkers and families.

A strong media partner can have a tremendous impact on a start-up race's success, and on its continued relevance over time. For Vancouverites, it's hard to imagine the Sun Run without the support of its eponymous newspaper. "The editorial staff and publisher really see the race as a twelve-month event," Gord added. "We post stories about participants and running and health clinics throughout the year. Staff writers who aren't runners will write about getting in shape to participate and how they launched their exercise program. Some have this picture of journalists as being cynical. But around this event, our people are very enthusiastic, year in, year out. We don't have to tell them to do so."

A favorite Sun Run memory for Gord came in 2013, the year of the Boston Marathon tragedy. "We wanted to make our event, which came within a few weeks of the bombing, a tribute to Boston," he recalled. "Though there were some concerns that people might be frightened to attend, we had a great turnout. I wore a Boston Bruins hockey jersey. The Bruins and our home team, the Canucks, are serious rivals. But I didn't hear a single boo."

GORD FISHER is president of the *National Post*, one of Canada's largest national daily newspapers, and also serves as president of Postmedia's Pacific Newspaper Group. Gord has an extensive media background and has held a number of senior executive positions in many Canadian cities on both the editorial and business sides of the media industry. He has previously served as publisher of the *National Post*, as well as president of the news and information division of Canwest Global Communications Corp.

If You Go

▶ **Getting There:** Vancouver is served by most major carriers.

▶ **Best Time to Visit:** The Vancouver Sun Run is held in late April. Vancouver's most reliably dry weather comes from June through September, though the route is generally snow-free throughout the year.

▶ **Race Information:** All the information you need about the Vancouver Sun Run resides at www.vancouversun.com/sunrun.

▶ **Accommodations:** The Hyatt Regency (888-591-1234; vancouver.regency.hyatt.com) serves as official race headquarters. Other lodging options are highlighted at Tourism Vancouver (604-682-2222; tourismvancouver.com).

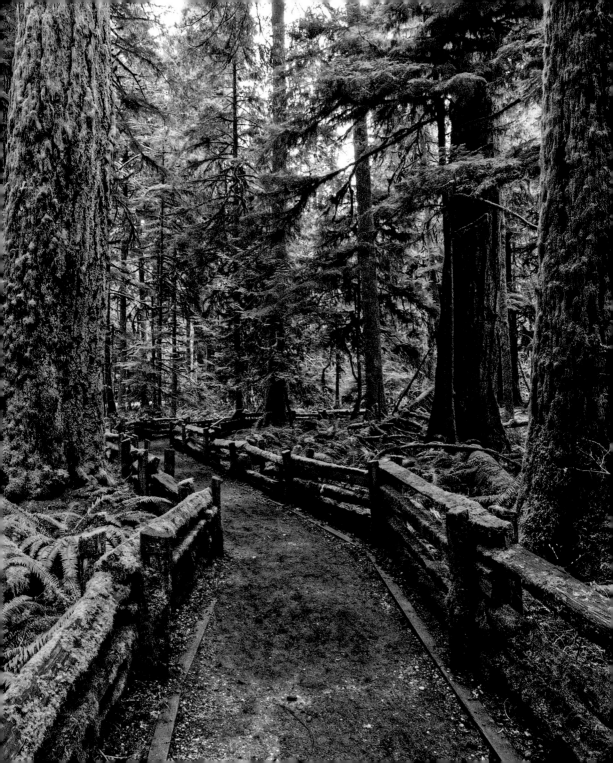

WEST COAST TRAIL

RECOMMENDED BY **Jen Segger**

Jen Segger has deep roots on Vancouver Island, so it's no great surprise that one of her favorite trail runs in the world is here—the West Coast Trail, in Pacific Rim National Park Reserve.

"Back in 2009, I took on something I called the Vancouver Island Quest," she began. "The goal was to traverse the whole island, north to south, a total of 466 miles, on foot. The idea was to link up trails, logging roads, mountain bike trails; I hoped to complete it in four days. I was running a lot at night to stay on schedule, and I was sleep deprived. By the time I got to the West Coast Trail, I was in the middle of this epic run, and it was hard to take everything in. All I really remember from the first run is that we missed the ferry crossing at the Nitinat River and had to spend the night huddled under rotting signs, with two space blankets for three people. At the time, I thought that I'd have to come back and do this when I'm fresh, and in the daylight."

Pacific Rim National Park Reserve is three parks in one, spread over 126,500 acres along the southwestern coast of Vancouver Island in British Columbia. It's composed of three units: the Long Beach unit, which has the most facilities and sees the most visitors; the Broken Group Islands unit, an archipelago of one hundred plus islands and islets scattered throughout Barkley Sound; and the West Coast Trail unit, a forty-seven-mile backpacking route through rain forests, along sandstone cliffs, and over beaches, from Bamfield to Port Renfrew. (The trail was once known as the Dominion Lifesaving Trail, because rescue workers would use it to reach shipwreck survivors along this rugged stretch of coastline.) This section of the park is home to some of North America's largest conifers, as well as some of the Pacific Rim's most notable creatures—cougars, wolves, and black bears. (The west coast of Vancouver Island has

OPPOSITE:
The West Coast Trail in Pacific Rim National Park Reserve passes old-growth forests, sandstone cliffs, and beaches.

the highest concentration of cougars in the world, but these secretive big cats are seldom seen . . . though it's likely *they will see you* as you make your way on the park's many trails through the forest.)

Hikers must commit to either the whole trail or half the trail, as there are only three access points. People covering the trail's entirety will often complete it in seven days. Endurance runners hope to conquer it in the course of a day.

Since her first experience on the West Coast Trail during her Vancouver Island Quest, Jen has covered the trail three times. "The second time, I took some runners from one of my coaching clients, Mountain Equipment Co-op," she continued. "They were 5K to 10K runners; I trained them up with the goal to conquer the trail. Once you reach a certain level of fitness, it's 90 percent mental. It was satisfying to watch these runners push themselves. They finished in under twenty-four hours. In the summer of 2015, my partner and I stand-up paddleboarded the length of the trail; we did it in three days and two nights, though we weren't trying for an FKT. In 2016, I wanted to go for an FKT on the trail."

There are a number of logistical considerations to address before setting off on the West Coast Trail. You must get a permit for using the trail and attend a mandatory trail orientation; coordinate a shuttle from the starting point to the ending point; and time your departure to make two ferry crossings (or be prepared to swim a small stretch of cold water at the run's conclusion). It's also helpful to time your departure for a day when there are low tides on the northern half of the trail, as this will allow you to run a long section of beach. Jen and her friends opted to run north to south, starting at five A.M. so they could make the ferry crossing at the Nitinat River by nine thirty, when the ferry starts to run.

"The trail starts out fairly easy in the woods, without much elevation gain," Jen described. "The tide was right for us to hit the beach. There was a lot of rock hopping, and that wasn't made any easier by the distraction of a pod of gray whales just off the beach. One of my favorite moments of the run comes toward the middle, as you approach Carmanah Lighthouse, one of the coast's iconic landmarks. You're on the beach, then you climb up all these steps, and the lighthouse is right there, surrounded by mowed green grass. It's a pinnacle point on the run; you can't help but think about all the shipwrecks when you're there. On this occasion, we barely made it, as the tide was coming up. But we stayed dry. From here, you drop down for a few kilometers and then reach Chez Monique. It's a little burger and beer stand in the middle of the wilderness, run by a feisty woman, Monique herself. Two of my fellow runners got twenty-dollar burgers, I got some butter tarts and Coke, and we pushed on. The terrain definitely gets tougher as you push on. I think the toughest stretch comes at the fifty-kilometer point—it's wet, muddy terrain with lots of exposed roots. It lasts about ten kilometers, and the mud always seems to be there, no matter how dry it's been. You just have to slog through."

Before the sun had set, Jen and her coconspirators had reached the Gordon River, with Port Renfrew looming beyond. They were prepared to brave the cold water and swim to the other shore, but luck was on their side. "We were starting to take off our socks and shoes and were waterproofing our packs," Jen said, "when a Zodiac came by. One of my friends jumped up and waved. The fisherman motored over and we offered him twenty dollars to bring us across, and he said, 'I don't want your money.' He was kind enough to take us across. We were able to make it to the Renfrew Pub before closing time, and soon we were toasting my women's FKT for the West Coast Trail—13:44:00 [down from a previous mark of 15:02:00]—with pints of cold Fat Tug IPA."

JEN SEGGER has been coaching athletes of all levels around the globe for more than a decade. Through a personalized approach, her athletes compete, participate, and achieve top results in ultra-running, mountaineering, Ironmans, triathlons, mountain bike races, road cycling, stand-up paddleboarding (SUP), and adventure races. Jen is an ACE personal trainer; USA Triathlon Level 1 coach; CrossFit Level I instructor; FaCT Level I tester; NCCP Triathlon Community Coach; YMCA Spin instructor; and Paddle Canada SUP instructor, River I & II. She also holds the female FKT for the Juan de Fuca Marine Trail (with Jenn Thiel)—forty-seven kilometers in seven hours, forty-nine minutes; and the female FKT for the Golden Hinde (with Sarah Seads)—fifty-three kilometers in nineteen hours, thirty-two minutes.

If You Go

▶ **Getting There:** Most visitors fly into Vancouver or Victoria and then drive to Pacific Rim (five hours from Victoria; 3.5 hours from Nanaimo, where the ferry from Vancouver

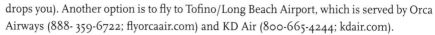

DESTINATION 6

drops you). Another option is to fly to Tofino/Long Beach Airport, which is served by Orca Airways (888- 359-6722; flyorcaair.com) and KD Air (800-665-4244; kdair.com).

▶ **Best Time to Visit:** The park is open from early May through mid-October; June through early September is the most popular time to visit.

▶ **Trail Information:** Parks Canada (250-726-3500; pc.gc.ca) has extensive information on the seventy-five-kilometer West Coast Trail, including how to apply for one of the limited number of permits. Given the trail's remote location, it's recommended that you run with a partner and use extreme caution if running at night. The six-mile stretch of Long Beach (in the park's first unit) is also popular with runners.

▶ **Accommodations:** In addition to camping options in the park, Vancouver Island Travel (vancouverisland.travel) highlights lodging options in Renfrew and near Bamfield.

BADWATER® 135 ULTRAMARATHON

RECOMMENDED BY **Chris Kostman**

Chris Kostman had been involved with endurance events in Death Valley for more than ten years before he took the reins of the Badwater® 135, considered by many to be the world's toughest footrace. "I'd first heard about the race around 1990 and was invited to participate in 1991," he recalled. "I ended up having to cancel, as the timing conflicted with a triathlon I was organizing in Canada. Not long after, I took on the management of an ultra-cycling event in Death Valley. I was intrigued that there was such a dramatic, desolate landscape in Southern California that so few people knew anything about. We did some cross-promotion of the cycling event and the Badwater 135. I ended up taking over the running event in 2000. At that point, it was really an underground race. There was no website, no media coverage, and no formal application process. The previous organizers weren't interested in considering athletes who couldn't speak English. I made a number of changes, including opening the event up to foreign participants, launching badwater.com, and developing the selection process. That first year, all six top finishers were from other countries, and now we average twenty countries represented each year. The Badwater 135 has become the de facto Olympics of endurance running events."

While there are races that have more elevation gain and descent, there are no events that have greater extremes in elevation levels or temperature than the Badwater 135 . . . and the distance certainly puts it in a class by itself. Beginning in Death Valley at Badwater Basin (282 feet below sea level and the lowest point in North America), the Badwater 135 winds its way west to its terminus at the Whitney Portal at 8,360 feet (which is the trailhead to Mount Whitney, the highest point in the contiguous United States at 14,505 feet). En route, it crosses three mountain ranges while gaining more than fifteen thousand feet in elevation. (The route is frequently bracketed by mountains reaching elevations of more

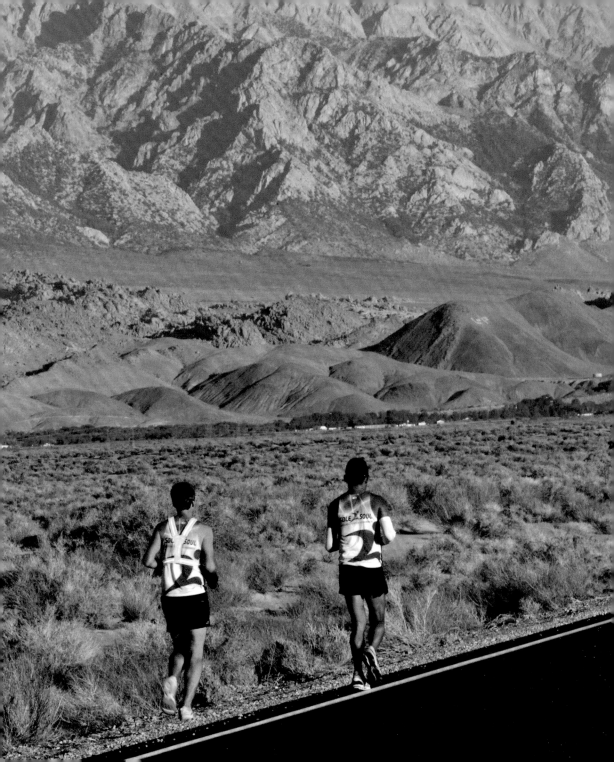

than eleven thousand feet.) To make what would be an amazing feat of endurance even more taxing, the Badwater 135 is held in July, when daytime temperatures can reach 120 degrees and nighttime temps can reach almost freezing at the finish line. Most of the hundred-odd runners who participate swathe themselves in white clothing to help reflect the relentless heat and protect them from sunburn. Since the air is warmer than your body, any breeze will increase your body temperature rather than decrease it, so complete coverage acts as insulation. (Acclimatizing to the heat is a key part of the preparation for the event; some will go as far as to run in a sauna.)

"One competitor, Frank McKinney, has called the Badwater 'running on the white line from hell to heaven,'" Chris continued. "You're going from the bowels of the hottest place on earth, where there's very little life, to mountains that are lush and green with an abundance of life. It's an incredible contrast. It's always so humbling to be out there in such an intense, dramatic landscape. It reminds you that we're just tiny little things in the blip of time."

The Badwater 135 route was first covered as a hike in 1969 by Jim Burnworth and Stan Rodefer. It was first run by Al Arnold, who's been called the "Edmund Hillary of ultramarathons." Al's first two attempts, in 1974 and 1975, were unsuccessful. But in 1977, he completed the course in roughly eighty hours . . . including the final segment on Whitney Portal Road, which climbs five thousand feet over thirteen miles. It was another ten years before the Badwater was organized as an official event. (In 2016, there were ninety-seven starters and eighty-four official finishers. As of this writing, the Badwater 135 men's record is 21:56:32, set by American Pete Kostelnick in 2016; the female record, 25:53:07, was established by American Alyson Venti in 2016.)

The race begins in the early evening. "Every year at the start, I announce, 'Whatever you do, don't think about the 135 miles of scorching desert terrain between here and the finish line,'" Chris said. "There's extreme variation along the whole route, and almost any kind of weather is possible. We've had rain, floods, wind- and sandstorms, even forest fires. Many are enamored with the ginormous sand dunes adjoining the road as you head into Stovepipe Wells. Towne Pass is also memorable—a seventeen-mile uphill, where you gain five thousand feet. Though it's not even halfway through, if runners can conquer this, they often feel they can finish. One thing that strikes you out there is the utter isolation of the place. It's seventeen miles before you reach the first intersection, another twenty-five miles to the next building, then eighty more before you reach anything faintly

OPPOSITE:
Extreme high
temperatures,
huge elevation
swings, and sheer
length make the
Badwater 135
Ultramarathon
one of America's
toughest
endurance races.

resembling civilization. I think of it as chasing the horizon. You'll see a landmark in the far distance, and it will take half a day to get there . . . and then you're on to the next horizon. Dean Karnazes won the Badwater in 2004. He likes to say that he didn't win, but 'survived it the fastest.'"

The extreme distance and conditions make setting up aid stations along the route impractical at best. "If we did, the volunteers might die," Chris said, only half-jokingly. Instead, each participant has a crew or support team (two to four members) that leapfrogs the runner along the course in a vehicle. "They'll provide food and water, spray runners to cool them down, deal with blisters, provide sunscreen and clothing changes," Chris explained. "It's almost as grueling as running, as you're jumping in and out of the car every mile or two. Most crews don't even bother running their air-conditioning. It's a team effort that gets each runner to the finish line."

Adversity can often breed camaraderie, and that certainly seems the case with the Badwater 135. "We could easily fill the race each year with veterans from previous races," Chris opined. "It becomes part of participants' identities. If they're not running, they're volunteering or serving on someone's crew. Three hundred of the same people are there every year. There's a sense of a Badwater family. Everyone is cheering for everybody else. People are constantly proving that human spirit and potential are limitless. We've had runners complete the race with prosthetic limbs. One runner—Art Webb—finished fourteen years in a row and got his best time the fourteenth year, at age seventy."

Chris will always recall an example of the Badwater spirit from 2009. "A man named Oswaldo Lopez had served on the support team for a winning racer named Jorge Pacheco," he shared. "In 2009, Oswaldo joined him in the race. Jorge was in the lead on the second big climb toward Lone Pine, but suddenly he wasn't feeling well. He went to rest in his support vehicle. Oswaldo approached. When he learned what was happening, he ran to the van and dragged Jorge out and told him, 'You've got to keep going. You've got to run with me.' At some races, the guy in second would blast by the leader. To see Oswaldo stop was just fantastic."

CHRIS KOSTMAN is the chief adventure officer at AdventureCORPS® Inc. and the race director of the Badwater Ultra Cup. He got his start early in ultra sports: He set world ultra-cycling records in high school in 1984 and 1985 (riding against the clock from San Francisco City Hall to Los Angeles City Hall) and completed the 3,127-mile, eleven-day

Race Across America bicycle race at age twenty in 1987. That was a springboard to competing in events as diverse as the Triple Ironman in France, the 6.5-mile Skaha Lake Ultra Swim in Canada, three hundred-mile snowshoe races in Alaska, and scores of twenty-four-hour mountain bike races and two-hundred-mile or longer road bike races. This led to a career producing some of the toughest endurance events available through his company, AdventureCORPS Inc. These include the world-famous Badwater 135 Ultramarathon footrace and its sister events, Badwater Salton Sea and Badwater Cape Fear, plus international events in China, Nepal, and Namibia. Chris has also published more than 250 articles about the endurance world. He is trained and educated as an archaeologist and works part-time in that field, both undersea and on land in the Middle East and South Asia. Learn more about Chris at chriskostman.com.

If You Go

▶ **Getting There:** Las Vegas is the closest major airport to both Furnace Creek and Lone Pine.

▶ **Best Time to Visit:** The STYR Labs Badwater 135 is held in mid-July each year.

▶ **Race Information:** The Badwater 135 accepts applications for the race in late January each year. A maximum of one hundred participants (who've completed at least three hundred-mile races) will be accepted. For details, visit badwater.com.

▶ **Accommodations:** Event planners block rooms at Furnace Creek Ranch (760-786-2345; furnacecreekresort.com) for before the event; several options are available in Lone Pine (near the finish line), including the Best Western Plus Frontier Motel (760-876-5571; bestwestern.com).

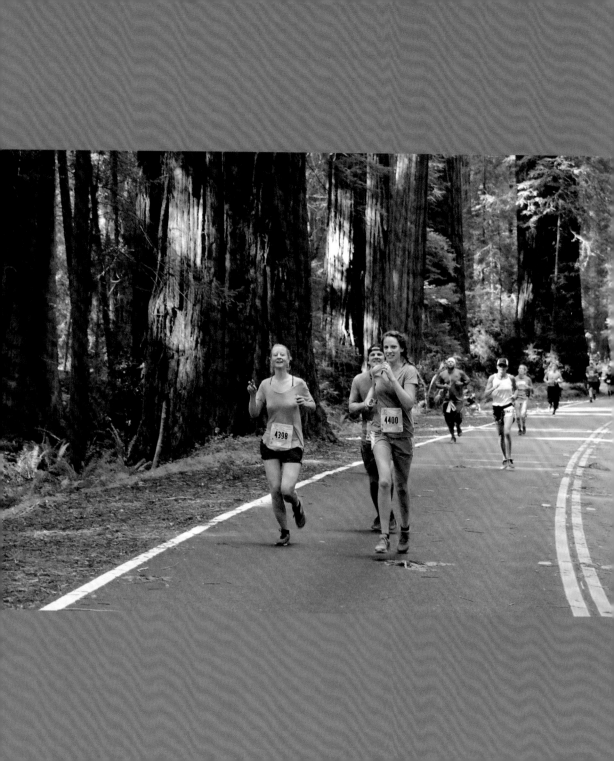

AVENUE OF THE GIANTS MARATHON

RECOMMENDED BY **Mairen Hughes**

In a time when many marathons have ballooned to tens of thousands of runners—begetting the need for ever greater sponsorships—the Avenue of the Giants Marathon has stayed small, eschewing corporate support. It may be because these runners in Northern California's Humboldt County don't need such bells and whistles . . . they have the trees of Humboldt Redwoods State Park.

"My very first marathon was the Rock 'n' Roll Marathon in Las Vegas," Mairen Hughes shared. "The crowds were a little overwhelming. The following spring, a friend said she was going to run the Avenue of the Giants and invited me to go. It's held in a very sparsely populated area. The towns nearby were small; everything seemed to be closed up at six o'clock! But the course was magnificent. It's basically a shorter and then a longer loop. The whole course is on pavement, but you're enveloped by the trees, so it feels like a trail run. It was so peaceful, I felt like I could let everything go."

The cool, moist climate of the north coast provides ideal conditions for coast redwoods (*Sequoia sempervirens*), the tallest known tree species in the world. Named for the reddish tone of their bark and heartwood, the largest specimens of coast redwoods can eclipse 350 feet in height and twenty feet in diameter; the average height ranges from 150 to 250 feet. The trees' thick bark, low resin content, and high levels of tannin foster strong resistance to disease, fire, and insects, helping make coast redwoods one of the longest-living tree species; some of the oldest specimens in Humboldt Redwoods State Park have been alive for more than two thousand years. (The park includes two other non-native redwood varieties—giant sequoias and dawn redwoods.) Redwoods have long been prized as lumber, and loggers began working the north coast as early as the 1850s, fueling the housing demands of San Francisco and other western cities.

OPPOSITE:
Avenue of
the Giants
in Humboldt
Redwoods State
Park showcases
some of America's
most majestic
forests.

The fact that the fifty-three-thousand-acre state park and its trees—the world's largest continuous old-growth redwood forest—exist is in part testimony to the efforts of three San Franciscans, John C. Merriam, Madison Grant, and Henry Fairfield Osborn. (Unfortunately, these men were also associated with the eugenics movement.) Having witnessed the devastation of the forests in southern Humboldt County during a trip north in 1917, the men founded the Save the Redwoods League. With the assistance of others in the community (including Laura Perott Mahan and the Humboldt County Women's Save the Redwoods League), they established Colonel Raynal C. Bolling Memorial Grove (which would later become the state park) just four years later. John D. Rockefeller visited the redwoods shortly thereafter and was impressed enough to donate several million dollars toward the purchase of additional land for preservation.

The idea of staging a marathon among the towering stands of redwoods emerged in early 1972, the brainchild of the Six Rivers Running Club. Local runners were seeking a nearby marathon that would give them a shot at qualifying for the 1972 US Olympic Trials. The state park fit the bill, with relatively flat topography, little traffic (especially in early May), and incomparable scenery. That first May, thirty-two runners left the starting line near Albee Creek Campground, and thirty of them finished. Though none qualified for the Olympic Games, American Frank Shorter's gold medal win for men's marathon triggered a nationwide interest in distance running. By 1977, more than one thousand entrants trekked to Humboldt County; to accommodate the increasing number of racers, the was course modified. Today, the event first loops alongside Bull Creek before following the South Fork of the Eel River on the Avenue of the Giants, which is a road as well as a park. (It was once part of Highway 101.) A 10K and half marathon were added over the years to offer less ambitious runners an opportunity to enjoy the serenity of a redwoods run.

"The weather was ideal for running during my visit," Mairen continued. "It was about sixty degrees and sunny, but the trees give you plenty of shade. I was very proud, as I was able to run the whole race, only stopping at the aid stations to rehydrate. My time for the Avenue of the Giants is still my personal best. At the end of the race there wasn't a big banquet, just a few food trucks—all very low-key. During the race, people were stopping to take pictures. I remember thinking, 'Why are they doing this?' Later, I wished I'd done the same. Those giant trees are so humbling."

While visiting Humboldt County, you may wish to take time to enjoy the redwoods at a slightly slower pace. Many like to visit the Dyerville Giant, a truly giant redwood that fell (of natural causes) in 1991. Arborists place its height at somewhere between 362 and 370 feet, taller than a thirty-story building. Its circumference at its base is fifty-two feet, and it's estimated to weigh more than one million pounds. If your legs have any spring left, consider a hike on Bull Creek Trail, which puts you in intimate contact with these noble trees. (The out-and-back northern portion is about 7.5 miles.) Be alert as you move quietly through these woods, as this is Bigfoot country—something you'll no doubt have noticed by the many Sasquatch bumper stickers, coffee cups, and other related paraphernalia you'll have encountered along Highway 101. No less of an authority than Cliff Barackman (founder of www.NorthAmericanBigfoot.com) has identified the redwoods of Humboldt County as an excellent place to go "bigfooting."

MAIREN HUGHES became interested in fitness after watching the Kona Ironman; she immediately registered for a triathlon, and her passion bloomed. She has competed in more than twenty races, including triathlons, duathlons, relays, and marathons. Mairen finds her motivation to push herself in fellow athletes and trainers who offer encouragement and support. As a fitness instructor, she has extended this encouragement to others who ask for help with their training, only to see them accomplish and exceed their goals. Mairen enjoys trail running, swimming, cycling, and rock climbing.

If You Go

▶ **Getting There:** The Avenue of the Giants is roughly a five-hour drive from San Francisco. The closest airport is near Eureka and is served by United (800-864-8331; united.com) and PenAir (800-448-4226; penair.com).

▶ **Best Time to Visit:** The Avenue of the Giants Marathon is held in early May. The road can be run throughout the year, though winters will inevitably be wet.

▶ **Race Information:** The Avenue of the Giants Marathon website (theave.org) lists race details, including registration information.

▶ **Accommodations:** The marathon website lists lodging options near the park. Garberville, twenty-five miles south of the starting line, has the most motel options.

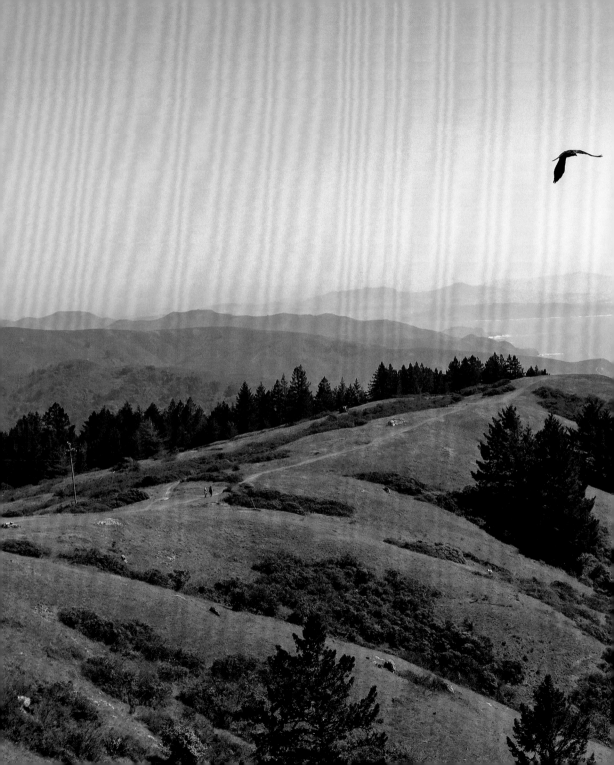

DIPSEA RACE

RECOMMENDED BY **Barry Spitz**

The Dipsea has the distinction of being the oldest trail race in America. For many, it's also one of the most special. Barry Spitz would place himself squarely in that camp. "I was the leading race announcer in America and have been involved in races all over. Between the spectacular nature of the course, its element of danger, and its handicap system, the Dipsea is special on many levels."

The 7.5-mile Dipsea Trail traverses the heart of Marin County, just north of San Francisco across the Golden Gate Bridge. It begins in downtown Mill Valley and ends at Stinson Beach, along the way gaining (and losing) 2,300 feet in elevation as you pass through Mount Tamalpais State Park, Muir Woods National Monument, the Golden Gate National Recreation Area, and a great deal of history . . . much of it on a narrow, steep single track. Barry details the Dipsea's pedigree on the race website as follows:

One summer day in 1904, several members of San Francisco's venerable Olympic Club set off for the Dipsea Inn, which had just opened on the Pacific Ocean sand spit now called Seadrift. They took the ferry to Sausalito, then the train to their starting point, the depot in Mill Valley. A wager was made as to who could make it to the inn first. The challenge proved so exciting that club members decided to make an annual race of it.

The next year, on a rainy November day, some one hundred runners participated in what the *San Francisco Examiner* would call "the greatest cross-country run that was ever held in this or any other country."

The Dipsea combines hiking trails, fire roads, and a few sections of macadam as runners make their way west to the Pacific. "Every section of the Dipsea Trail has a name

OPPOSITE:
Cardiac Hill, the
highest point on
the iconic Dipsea
Race route.

and some lore attached," Barry continued. "The race starts in Lytton Square, named after Mill Valley's first resident, and soon you reach the Dipsea Steps—688 right now [broken into three sets]. I can't think of any other race that has an obstacle like this so early; everyone who does the race talks about the steps. The trail continues to climb until you hit your first crest at Windy Gap. Then there's a steep plunge down Muir Woods Road into the Muir Woods valley. From here, you have your second big climb up a section called Dynamite as you're surrounded by deep redwood forest. You come out on a hogback of grassland that was once used to graze cows. Then you enter a section called the Rainforest, an area of virgin redwoods that have been preserved for many years, and start to climb. The crest on that climb is called Cardiac Hill, which should give you an idea of its difficulty. Next is a short, level stretch of trail—one of few on the course—named Baron's Rest. Now you start the plunge down. There's the Swoop, which I'd call very dangerous, and Steep Ravine, a series of something like four hundred steps that I'd call incredibly dangerous. How people go down at all at speed, much less passing people, I don't understand. People break bones here all the time. After Steep Ravine, you get a glimpse of the ocean. It gets you going, but there's another mile to go. Once runners reach Stinson Beach, some will go into the ocean. There's a good deal of poison oak on the trail, and some people think the salt water will help wash it off. I'm not sure if it does any good.

"I've done a lot of award ceremonies in my day, and most of the time maybe half of the people who win stick around. But that's not the case at the Dipsea. All thirty-five people who win stick around to get black numbered shirts. That black shirt is special."

The Dipsea's handicap system is another unique facet of the race. "Originally, runners got a head start based on their ability," Barry explained. "In that setting, everyone at the starting line felt they had a chance to win. But as the field grew, there were too many runners, so the handicapping changed to be based first on age, then on gender. In this setting, the best runners in each age group have the best chance of winning. The system has produced winners ranging from eight-year-old girls to seventy-two-year-old men."

For Barry, one of the Dipsea's most endearing qualities is how deeply it has woven its way into the lives of so many participants. "The first winner was a high school student named John Hassard," he recalled. "John didn't have children, but his siblings did, and Hassards are still running the race today. When I was writing the history of the Dipsea, I spoke to a woman who's in her nineties. It turns out that her mother won the Dipsea women's hike in 1919. (It should be noted that the Dipsea had events for women when few other venues did.) One of my favorite stories concerns Norman Bright. He ran for Stanford in the 1930s, and in 1937, he broke the course record, which had held since 1912. Norm came back many years later, with his sight failing. His record was still standing. He was sixty, and he hoped to break the sixty-minute mark. He ran the course in fifty-nine something . . . and the next finisher broke his course record.

"People have a long-term commitment to this race."

BARRY SPITZ has been the Dipsea Race finish line and awards ceremony announcer since 1982 and the race's official historian since 1993. As a volunteer he has never been able to run the race, but he's completed more than twenty Practice Dipsea, Double Dipsea, and Quadruple Dipsea races. A longtime runner, Barry has logged some seventy-five thousand miles and has been a member of the Tamalpa Runners since 1978. He is the author of seven history and outdoor books, including *Dipsea: The Greatest Race*. Since 1989, he has written a weekly column on running for the *Marin Independent Journal*. Barry also leads hikes in the region. He is particularly proud of receiving the James Farren Jr. Trophy for "sportsmanship, leadership, and dedication to the race" in 1992, the Dipsea's Jerry Hauke Trophy in 2002, and a Milley Award in 2001. Learn more about Barry at dipseabook.com.

If You Go

▶ **Getting There:** San Francisco is served by most major carriers.
▶ **Best Time to Visit:** The Dipsea Race is held the second Sunday in June, but most of the course can be run year-round.
▶ **Race Information:** Detailed information resides at the Dipsea Race website (dipsea.org). Competition for a slot is rigorous; more than 3,000 people apply for the 1,500 spots.
▶ **Accommodations:** The Marin Convention and Visitors Bureau (866-925-2060; visit marin.org) lists lodging options in Mill Valley and Marin County.

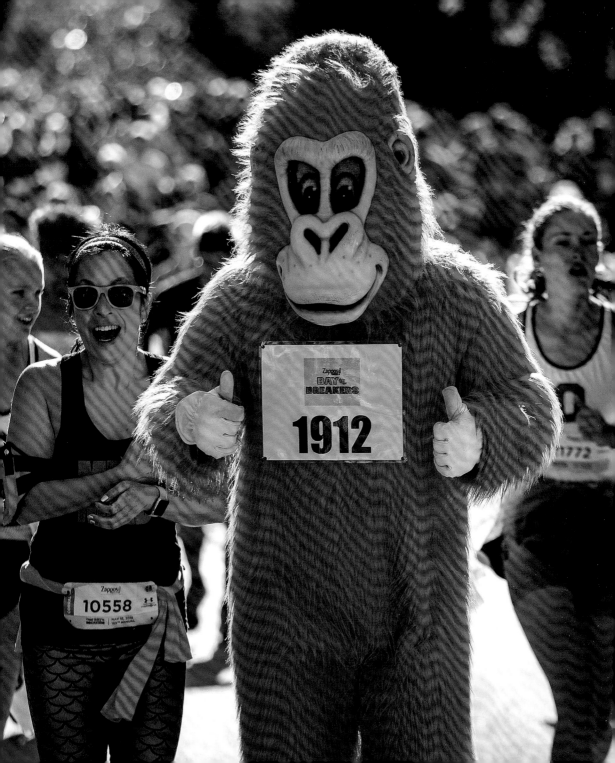

BAY TO BREAKERS

RECOMMENDED BY **Chris Holmes**

San Francisco has always been the kind of open and accepting city where people can go to be who they want to be. While skyrocketing rents and an increasing gap between the wealthy and the poor have no doubt changed the complexion of the City by the Bay, there's at least one time of year when people can come to San Francisco and let their freak flag fly—the running of the Bay to Breakers each May.

Chris Holmes fondly recalls his first experience with the Bay to Breakers. "I got my first taste of the race just after college. I was living in Los Angeles but had friends in San Francisco. One of them called and said, 'You have to come up for this race.' I asked him to tell me what it was about, and he said, 'I can't explain it. Just come . . . and dress as Super Mario.' I did, and had an incredible time. I ran it a few more times over the next ten years and then had the chance to take over the race's management. Knowing what a great event it was, I was eager to do so. It's an event that works on several levels. For more traditional runners it's a bucket list event, thanks to the visual pleasure of the course. It showcases San Francisco in so many ways, taking you past iconic landmarks like the Painted Ladies, Golden Gate Park, and Ocean Beach. Runners are also drawn to the Bay to Breakers for the distance. At twelve kilometers, it's a bit odd, and it intrigues people who've done a 5K, 10K, or half marathon. For more casual runners or walkers, it's an excuse to gather some friends together and put on a crazy costume."

Given the race's somewhat whimsical nature, many are surprised to learn that the Bay to Breakers dates back more than one hundred years—though in its initial incarnation, it was a bit more traditional. The first event—then known as the Cross City Race—was held in 1912 and had 186 participants. (The race was initiated in part by city fathers to elevate the morale of San Franciscans after the devastation of the 1906 earthquake.) Some

OPPOSITE:
Imaginative
costumes are as
much a part of
Bay to Breakers
as the great vistas
of San Francisco's
landmarks.

seventy years later, the Bay to Breakers set a Guinness World Record as the planet's biggest running event, with 110,000 participants. (In recent years, it's attracted a more modest field of fifty-thousand-plus runners, and more than one hundred thousand spectators.) While the course has evolved over time, the basic premise has remained the same: Runners begin on the east side of the city near the shores of San Francisco Bay and conclude 7.5 miles later at San Francisco's western boundary, where the Pacific laps at Ocean Beach.

The chance to run through one of America's most beautiful cities is one distinguishing facet of the Bay to Breakers. But for many, the event is defined by its costumes. Most agree that the first costumed runner was dressed as a pirate named Captain Kidd and participated in 1940. The captain's costume initiative didn't take off immediately. More costumed runners began appearing in the 1970s and '80s, but the tradition really became a cornerstone in 1992, when race organizers sponsored the first costume contest. "I'm amazed at the detail and the amount of time spent on costumes each year," Chris continued. "There are some guys who spend six dollars at the thrift store the day before, but there are others who spend months. The tandem costumes are the most intriguing to me. My favorite is a full replica of the Golden Gate Bridge, carried by two people, each with a tower on their shoulder. It's hard to fathom how they can keep it together." A perennial favorite among spectators is a group of runners dressed as salmon, who run the race-course in reverse, as though swimming upstream.

Another defining characteristic of the Bay to Breakers is the presence of linked runners, or centipede teams. Centipede teams are groups of at least thirteen runners who must run linked together by a bungee cord or other safe means throughout the race . . . and often in themed costume. The centipede tradition was pioneered by members of the UC Davis Track Club in 1978. "This past year, there was a women's centipede team dressed as snow globes," Chris recalled. "Each globe depicted a different city around the world—Paris, Las Vegas, New York. The first year I ran it, I was part of a centipede team; we were all Mario Brothers characters." While many centipedes are in it for fun, there are serious runners too: The winning team in 2016 took places twenty-three to thirty-five. (If you find yourself near the six-mile mark on the course, be on the lookout for centipedes performing the infamous Lenichi Turn . . . a mythical maneuver you'll have to see for yourself!)

There is certainly a good deal of frivolity associated with the Bay to Breakers. At one point, the festivities accompanying the race almost threatened its future. "Some years back, the partying had gotten out of hand, and city officials considered canceling the event," Chris shared. "But people were able to rein things in and still keep it a fun event. We've been working to put the focus back on the run itself." And the course is no push-over. "The section of the run that everyone talks about is the Hayes Street Hill," Chris continued. "It's a beast from the bottom to Alamo Square—two-thirds of a mile with a 14 percent grade. People often think that all is fine after Hayes, but there's a subtle incline that extends for two miles as you head west on Fell Street into Golden Gate Park. You can't really see it, but it zaps you. But when you're halfway through the park, you hit a downslope that takes you all the way to the ocean."

And this being San Francisco, a great party with a beer garden and live music awaits at the finish line.

CHRIS HOLMES is vice president of endurance at Wasserman, a full-service sports marketing and talent management agency that serves the best athletes, brands, and properties in the world.

If You Go

- **Getting There:** San Francisco is served by most major carriers.
- **Best Time to Visit:** The Bay to Breakers race is held the third Sunday in May.
- **Race Information:** Everything you need to know about the Bay to Breakers (including registration information) can be found at baytobreakers.com, or by calling 415-231-3130.
- **Accommodations:** The official hotel for the event is the Hyatt Regency (415-788-1234; sanfrancisco.regency.hyatt.com). The San Francisco Convention and Visitors Bureau (415-974-6900; sfvisitor.org) highlights other options.

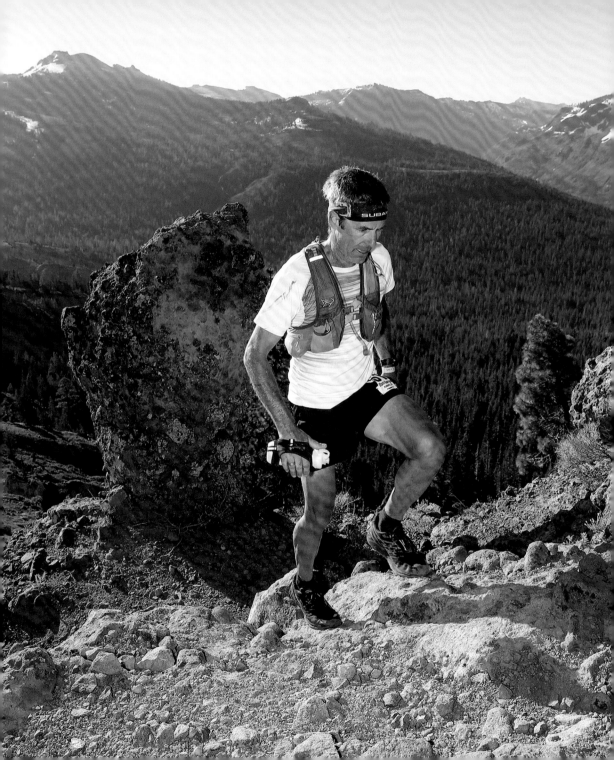

WESTERN STATES®

100-MILE ENDURANCE RUN

RECOMMENDED BY **Tim Twietmeyer**

The Western States® 100-Mile Endurance Run is the great granddaddy of endurance runs, dating back to 1974. "It's the original hundred-miler," Tim Twietmeyer began. "The way marathoners strive to one day compete in the Boston Marathon, endurance runners hope to come to the Sierras to see what they can do . . . and if they can break the twenty-four-hour mark. The Western States Trail dates back to the pioneer days. There were other trails that took you over the mountains, but the Western States was the most direct. It's also the hardest."

And that's the trail that's run.

The course for the Western States 100-Mile Endurance Run begins in Squaw Valley (near the town of Tahoe City) and runs 100.2 miles west to its terminus in the town of Auburn. (The complete trail actually begins in Salt Lake City and ends in Sacramento.) Along the way it gains more than eighteen thousand feet in elevation and drops nearly twenty-three thousand feet; climbs more than passes that reach nearly nine thousand feet; demands the fording of an icy-cold river; and follows the wagon ruts of miners who once heeded the clarion call of gold and silver echoing from the Sierra foothills. Much of the trail traverses rugged, remote mountain and canyon terrain that, while beautiful, can be unforgiving. Potentially violent temperature swings (from lows of 20 degrees in the mountains to highs of 105 in the valley) add to the challenge. (The event's website offers many cautions for the uninitiated.)

The Western States has equestrian roots. In 1955, a group of six horsemen led by Wendell T. Robie set out to prove that horses could still cover one hundred miles in one day. They succeeded, and an annual ride, known as the Tevis Cup, was soon established. In 1974, a rider named Gordy Ainsleigh, who had already completed the course on

OPPOSITE:
A runner
approaches
Cougar Rock,
one of the
toughest
climbs on the
Western States
Endurance Run.

59

horseback, decided to see if he could match the performance of the horses with his own two legs. He did it, with eighteen minutes to spare. In 1977, the first official running event was held, with fourteen participants and three finishers. In the early days, it was determined that those who completed the course in less than twenty-four hours would receive a handmade silver belt buckle commemorating their achievement; those who finished in less than thirty hours, the race's cutoff time, would receive a bronze buckle. Both bear the likeness of a mountain lion. (In 2016, there were 353 starters and 280 finishers.)

The course has had a few alterations over the years and occasionally must be tweaked thanks to lingering snow. But the core elements remain intact. Tim described a few of the highlights. "To me, the trail has three distinct zones. The first thirty miles, you're in alpine terrain, above six thousand feet, and you're running big ridges and river drainages. The middle section is all about running canyons; this is where a lot of people start to fall apart. At the forty-six-mile point, there's a steep climb to a spot called Devil's Thumb. When first-timers hit it, the math is not panning out. You're not quite halfway but seem to have spent 85 percent of your energy. To make matters worse, it's the hottest part of the day, and some of the trail is exposed to the sun. In the end, you're in the foothills, running through grasslands, manzanita, and oak. I think this is the best running. Except for a mile near the middle and a mile or so at the end, you're all on dirt. On the middle section, around Last Chance and Michigan Bluff, you're running over all kinds of mining history—abandoned shafts, buildings, and graveyards. It's quiet now, but it must have been pretty crazy then, in the 1850s. A great landmark near the end is No Hands Bridge, a cement arch built in 1912. It didn't used to have guardrails, but now it does so no one goes over the side."

The very fastest competitors can minimize the time spent running at night, but most everyone covering the trail will experience at least a portion of it in darkness. This is an experience in itself. "Everything slows down," Tim described, "and all you can see is fifteen or twenty feet ahead. If you haven't done the course before, you're not sure what's coming. Sometimes you'll see lights way ahead or way back. Some weird critters are coming out—snakes, raccoons, skunks. It's very surreal. Your senses are so much more alert at the end, even though you're super tired, as you have to rely on something other than vision." Runners can opt to have a pacer accompany them for the night portion of the race, to help them stay on course and run safely.

Tim has the distinction of having won the Western States not once, not twice, but five times (with more than twenty-five sub-twenty-four-hour finishes). His memories of his first time competing—and of his first victory—still resonate. "I first ran the Western States in 1981. There was no Internet, of course, so I had no course knowledge. Finishing that first time was a life-changing experience. As you're running, you don't know if you'll make it, how deep you'll need to dig. Over the next ten years, I finished in the top ten, even the top five a few times. I couldn't help but begin to wonder if I was ever going to break through. But in 1992, I did. It was a bit like Bill Rodgers winning the Boston Marathon. It was never really my goal to win, but by working hard at it I made it. When I was competing, there were two people I learned from—Dick Collins and Ruth Anderson. Neither was particularly fast, but their lesson was in how they conducted themselves on the trail. They showed me that you're competing *with* someone, rather than against.

"An event like the Western States is curious. You prepare for six months, run it in twenty-four hours . . . and then talk about it for six months. Some will say, 'I'll never do it again.' But then you start thinking that if you spent a little less time at that one aid station, you could probably cut twenty minutes off your time. And you think about signing up again."

TIM TWIETMEYER first ran the Western States 100 at only twenty-two years of age, a feat that he returned to complete twenty-four more times, all with impressive sub-twenty-four-hour finishes. He was also the first man to win five Western States, winning in 1992, 1994–1996, and 1998, and has previously held the course record with a time of 17:17:00 in the masters (over forty years of age) division. Tim has completed more than two hundred marathon and ultramarathon races during his career. He has completed the American River 50 Mile Run and the California International Marathon more than twenty times each and has won the California 50-Mile Endurance Run seven times. Tim's fifty-mile and 50K wins are too numerous to mention. He has also won the Eagle 100 in Canada and has completed the Ultra-Trail du Mont-Blanc, the most difficult trail race in Europe. Tim's fastpacking accomplishments include a sub-six-day completion of the 211-mile John Muir Trail and the first completion of the 165-mile Tahoe Rim Trail in less than two days. When not out running or competing, Tim spends his time with his wife and three sons. He has served twenty years on the board of trustees of the Western States Endurance Run Foundation, including five years as president.

If You Go

▶ **Getting There:** The closest airport to Tahoe City is in Reno; the closest airport to Auburn is in Sacramento. Both are served by most major domestic carriers.

▶ **Best Time to Visit:** The Western States 100-Mile Endurance Run takes place on the last weekend in June each year.

▶ **Race Information:** The Western States website (wser.org) highlights all elements of the race, including the entry process. Entrants who've completed a qualifying event are entered in a lottery; from this lottery, 369 participants are chosen.

▶ **Accommodations:** The North Lake Tahoe website (gotahoenorth.com) highlights lodging options near the race's start. Placer County Visitors Bureau (866-752-2371; visitplacer.com) lists options near the finish line.

CONQUER THE WALL MARATHON

RECOMMENDED BY **Mosi Smith**

For more than two thousand years, the Great Wall has stood as a psychological—if not a physical—barrier between China and the rest of the world. Since 1999, it has been repurposed—at least in small part—as a running course.

And what a running course!

Mosi Smith shared how he came to experience the Great Wall. "I had just transitioned from active duty military," he recalled. "I did some traveling around the world, and was back home in Maryland for a brief period, figuring out my next adventure. I logged on to Facebook, and there was a notice looking for some people to measure and recon some courses in China. I got in touch with the organizers, and I met all the criteria they needed. I was thrilled, as I grew up thinking about the Great Wall. As a runner, I couldn't help but think how cool it would be to see this historical place and run right beside it . . . or even on it. I traveled there to help establish the courses for the coming year, and the landscape far exceeded my expectations. Unfortunately, life got busy for a few years, and I missed the opportunity to run the race that spring. Eventually, I was able to go and take on the challenge firsthand. People often ask, 'What's your toughest marathon?' Removing temperature extremes, it is the Conquer the Wall Marathon. There's the jet lag (at least if you're coming from the States); you're at a smidge of elevation, just enough to question if you've done enough training; it gets pretty hot, and with the exception of a few spots where you're in the shadow of towers or trees, you're exposed. The steps are the quiet little hitters. If you run a full marathon out there, you're going to feel like you've run twice as long. If you want a predictor for a time, anticipate taking two and a quarter times your normal marathon pace."

The Great Wall of China has been a work in progress for much of its existence. Though imperfect and in slow demise (thanks to minimal maintenance), the wall—

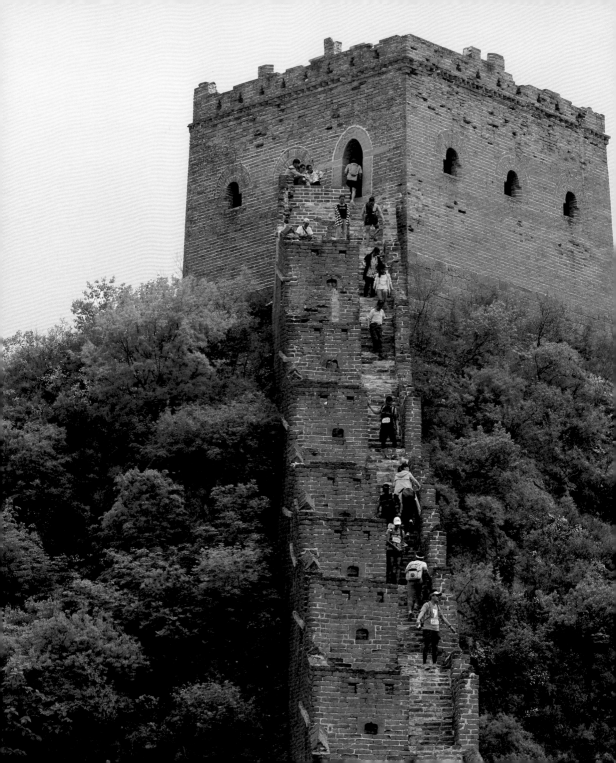

known in China as the Long Wall of Ten Thousand Li—still stands as one of the world's great construction achievements. (It might be more accurate to think of it as a long series of smaller walls and other fortifications, rather than one monolithic structure.) Though it was first imagined in the third century BCE by Emperor Qin Shi Huang, the sections of the wall that are best known (and in the best condition) were constructed during the Ming dynasty, between the fourteenth and seventeenth centuries. The most popular section of the Great Wall for visitors is around Badaling, which is fifty miles northwest of Beijing.

The Conquer the Wall Marathon takes place in the Badaling region—slightly removed from the busiest tourist sections. (Another event, the Great Wall Marathon [operated by Albatros Adventure Marathons], is run along the Huangyaguan Great Wall, roughly eighty miles east of Beijing.) "One aspect of the event that people should be aware of is that it's almost more of an adventure trail run," Mosi continued. "I imagined that the wall would be a bit more built-up, but many portions are very degraded, with the government working to make steady repairs and improvements each year. Parts of the course are simply a path along the spine of a ridge with bricks here or there. [The race program mentions that on the course, 'You'll encounter loose stones, gravel, missing steps, and crumbling walls along with trees and grass in some areas.'] But when you do get to a spot where the wall has been restored, you're encountering something that's like a stair workout on crack." Not all of the course is on or alongside the Great Wall, it should be noted. There are loops that take runners through several small villages before returning to the wall.

About those steps: Depending on the section of the wall that is run, there are between ten thousand and twenty thousand countable steps along the length of the race. For runners, it seems that no two are the same. "The vertical differential between sets varies from two inches to two-plus feet," Mosi explained. "They were engineered this way intentionally to slow down invading forces. Dealing with the deviations in the steps precludes ease of foot movement and the establishment of a rhythm during a skirmish."

Assembling a marathon anywhere poses certain logistical challenges; doing so in the Chinese countryside only increases the number of potential impasses. But Mosi was impressed with how smoothly things unfolded. "The organizers did a great job planning for the unknown and pulling together surrounding communities," Mosi said. "Still, I

OPPOSITE:
Steep, uneven
steps are among
the obstacles that
make Conquer
the Wall seem
like running two
marathons.

think it's good to go into such an event with the capacity to be self-sustaining. Additionally, I was a bit concerned that a large footprint of runners had potential to damage this great cultural site. But the section of the course we ran was well chosen. I would say that the organizers have been good stewards of the wall."

It's safe to say that marathons are not yet a big spectator sport in rural China. "For the most part, the only committed spectators were there to support individual entrants," Mosi recalled. "We did come upon tourists on a few occasions, and a few would post up around the towers on the wall and cheer runners on. When the loops took us into the villages, the people were very inquisitive. It seemed that they'd gotten the gist of what was going on, and they'd give a 'hello.'

"Overall, the experience of running on the Great Wall was completely surreal. Every mile or so I'd have to stop, look around, and take a photo. I had to remind myself that people don't often have a chance to do this. One of the moments I recall came when we were returning to the wall after one of the village loops. The course took us up a small hill, then you'd mount the wall. The first couple hundred yards were very steep, maybe thirty degrees. I could see a trail of people ahead, and as I climbed, I was trying to be mindful of not kicking rocks down on the runners behind me. We all worked hard to get to the top of that climb. And we all paused to appreciate the moment."

MOSI SMITH is a veteran and officer in the US Marine Corps. He has been an avid runner since 1996. He is a certified coach through USA Track & Field and the Road Runners Club of America, and was the assistant coach of the US Naval Academy Marathon Team. Mosi has completed eighty-one marathons and longer-distance runs, including the Boston Marathon (six times), Ironman Triathlons, the Western States® 100, the Marathon des Sables, and the Badwater® 135 Ultramarathon. He is the race director of the Annapolis Striders' Endless Summer 6-Hour Run in Annapolis, Maryland, benefiting the Semper Fi Fund, which has raised more than $25,000 for the organization. Life post–Marine Corps for Mosi has included working in the outdoor retail and event management industry, traveling to support friends in their athletic pursuits, feeding his spirit of wanderlust, and becoming a stronger athlete and a better person.

If You Go

▶ **Getting There:** Most visitors will fly into Beijing, which is served by most international carriers.

▶ **Best Time to Visit:** The various marathons conducted on and near the Great Wall of China are held in May.

▶ **Race Information:** Details and registration information for the Conquer the Wall Marathon resides at conquerthewallmarathon.com. Information about the Great Wall Marathon can be found at great-wall-marathon.com.

▶ **Accommodations:** The Renaissance Beijing Capital Hotel (+86 1058638888; marriott.com/hotels/travel/bjsbc-renaissance-beijing-capital-hotel) is race headquarters. Transportation to the race site in Badaling is provided.

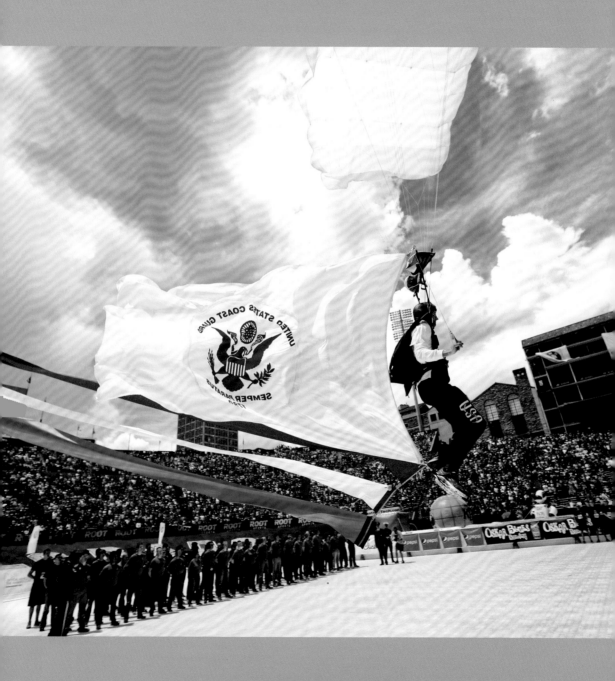

BOLDERBOULDER

RECOMMENDED BY **Cliff Bosley**

As many residents of Boulder, Colorado, will readily tell you, the home of the University of Colorado Golden Buffaloes rests at an elevation of 5,350 feet. This elevation—and Boulder's proximity to the Rockies—has fostered a culture steeped in endurance sports and outdoor activities. Many elite athletes—skiers, runners, bikers, rock climbers—choose to train here, and that in turn has spawned many businesses to serve the outdoor and fitness community. A popular T-shirt here reads "Sea Level Is for Sissies." The words "BolderBOULDER" are printed on the sleeve . . . and the race seems to encapsulate what the town is all about.

"The BolderBOULDER began in 1979, when I was twelve," Cliff Bosley recalled. "My dad founded the event. He'd taken up jogging in the late sixties after his dad died at age sixty from a heart attack. In the late seventies, my siblings and I were involved in track; the race was initially conceived as a track meet for kids. Frank Shorter [winner of the gold medal in the men's marathon at the 1972 Summer Olympics] lived in Boulder then (and still does), and my dad asked if he'd get involved. After the second meeting, Frank said, 'Putting together a track meet will be pretty complicated. How about a road race?' My dad said, 'What's a road race?' But pretty soon he visited a few, and the first iteration of the BolderBOULDER came together. My Boy Scout troop was tasked with promoting the event. We went door to door with posters that said 'Race against Frank Shorter and Ric Rojas' [Rojas was ranked among the top ten US road racers by *Track & Field News* from 1977 to 1981]. Pro athletes were central to the successful promotion of running at that time, and with Frank's help, my dad had early success in getting world-class athletes to come to Boulder. To this day, the professional heats of the BolderBOULDER remain a priority. But our biggest message has been one of inclusivity, to get lots of people out

OPPOSITE:
Skydivers with
service flags
representing each
branch of the
military service
cap off the Bolder
BOULDER
at Folsom
Field, run each
Memorial Day.

running. The battle cry from the outset has been 'Oh Yes You Can!' This means different things to different people. For some, it means you can get a personal best. For others, it means you can run the course without stopping. For us, it was always an invitation for people to come out and run—or walk—ten thousand meters. That's how we still think about it today."

The BolderBOULDER unfolds for 6.2 miles through the rolling hills of the city, show-casing the Flatirons (an iconic rock formation), the town, and the university along the way. "There's plenty of entertainment along the course," Cliff continued. "Every 250 to 300 yards, there's a garage band, Elvises, belly dancers, spectators offering bacon, marsh-mallows, watermelon. In recent years, someone set up a Slip 'N Slide near the midpoint. Hundreds take advantage. As much as it's a serious event, there are whimsical elements too." Over the years, the course has had nine iterations. "The first year, the race had 2,700 participants, and it concluded at a park in north Boulder," Cliff recalled. "The next year, the field expanded to five thousand and finished at Boulder High on their football field. Before the third race, the president and the athletic director of the University of Colorado came to see my father. They said that the BolderBOULDER has gotten to be a big deal—it should finish at the University of Colorado. Ever since, the finish line has been at Folsom Field." The thrill of entering a stadium with fifty thousand (or more) fans cheering you on—whether your time is thirty-eight minutes or two hours and thirty-eight minutes—is a special appeal of the race.

One of the BolderBOULDER's claims to fame has been the wave start, which the event pioneered in 1984 and has been fine-tuning ever since. "We have almost one hundred different start groups now for more than fifty thousand participants, from qualifying elites to walkers," Cliff described. "This setup of staggered starts creates an opportunity for everyone to do their best run. We don't have a cap on the event, and I like that. I want everyone who wishes to participate to be able to be part of this experience." Though a broad part of the running public participates in the BolderBOULDER, the event is marked by a fast field; 2016 had six hundred finishers who broke the forty-minute mark; Atlanta, where the elevation is about one thousand feet above sea level, had three hundred sub-forty finishers in the Peachtree 10K.

Late morning, when the last amateur participants have entered the stadium, the pro-fessional running race begins. (A pro wheelchair race is conducted before the waves begin.) Runners from around the world compete for one of the largest non-marathon purses. The event is televised live on large screens in the stadium. An added twist is the International Team Challenge. The top three runners from each participating country are scored cross-country style; the team with the lowest score is the winner.

The BolderBOULDER is held each May on Memorial Day, and once the running has concluded, the event takes time to honor the men and women of the armed services. "We see this as a unique opportunity to recognize each branch of the military," Cliff said. "In the twenty-five-minute program, we have skydivers with service flags for each branch, plus one for POWs and one carrying an American flag. There's an F-16 flyover and a chance for some veterans to tell their unique stories. We usually have seventy-five thousand people in attendance."

There are sixty-two people who have run every BolderBOULDER. This group—known as the BolderBOULDER's Boldest (BBB)—includes Cliff's younger brother Ted. When asked why he wasn't a BBB member, Cliff explained, "The third year of the race, I was offered a spot on the press truck to help photograph the race. For a fourteen-year-old, that was a pretty unique opportunity to act in an official capacity. Frank Shorter was a hero of mine, and he won the race that year. Having grown up around this race, having volunteered for it and run it, I've felt very privileged to be involved in something that brings our community together and touches them. There have been so many special moments. But documenting Frank's victory is certainly near the top."

CLIFF BOSLEY is the race director of the BolderBOULDER.

If You Go

▶ **Getting There:** Most visitors to Boulder will fly into Denver, which is served by most major carriers.
▶ **Best Time to Visit:** The BolderBOULDER is held in late May, on Memorial Day.
▶ **Race Information:** In-depth information (including registration) can be found at bb10k.bolderboulder.com.
▶ **Accommodations:** The Boulder Convention & Visitors Bureau (303-442-2911; bouldercoloradousa.com) lists a host of lodging options.

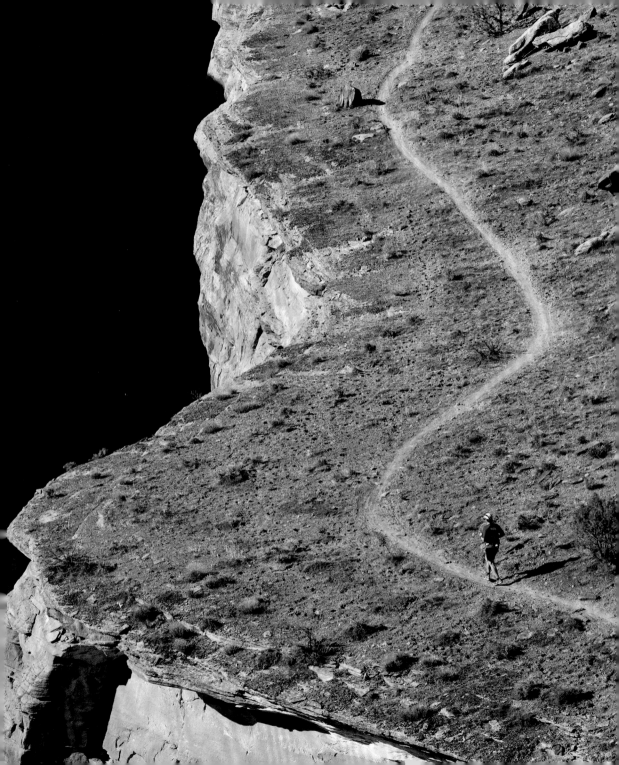

DESERT RATS TRAIL RUNNING FESTIVAL

RECOMMENDED BY **Reid Delman**

Those familiar with the western Colorado communities of Fruita and Grand Junction know them for their epic mountain biking trails. The Kokopelli Trail system—some 140 miles of tracks that stretch west to Moab, Utah—includes some of the sport's most storied terrain, skirting arid canyons along the mighty Colorado River. Reid Delman knew the regional trails' fat tire appeals . . . but he imagined something else.

"It was in the early 2000s, and bad weather had canceled a popular trail race in western Colorado," Reid recalled. "I knew there were amazing mountain biking trails around Fruita. I thought I'd try to put on some running races that follow some of the same trails—loop courses, but with different distances. Once we got people out on the trails, the trails sold themselves. I live on the east side of the mountains, but I love the desert—the open spaces and dry air. By creating a weekend of events with the Desert RATS Trail Running Festival, we were hoping to foster a celebration of the area and its fantastic trails. It's safe to say that it was the trails that got me started, but it's the people that keep me doing this. Ultra-runners are a different breed."

Fruita is situated in far western Colorado, tucked between the small city of Grand Junction and the Utah border. The Colorado River flows south of the town, which is bracketed by the Book Cliffs to the north. This area of western Colorado is a far cry from the lushly forested alpine regions like Aspen and Vail. This is mesa and canyon country, a land of open spaces and little precipitation (less than ten inches of rain a year). This wide-open country makes for some big views. As its name implies, Fruita was first established as a fruit-growing region, back in the 1880s. Initially, apples were cultivated; later, peaches, pears, and cherries. In more recent years, Fruita has undergone a rebranding of sorts, evolving into an outdoor recreational hot spot. (If you're a fan of avian anomalies,

OPPOSITE:
A lone run-
ner near a cliff
edge above the
Colorado River
during the Desert
RATS Trail
Running Festival.

73

sideshows, or both, you might recall that Fruita was once home of Mike the Headless Chicken. After a botched butchering, the rooster in question lived on for eighteen months sans head, with his owner feeding him grain and water through his neck with an eyedropper; though his head had been severed, his brain stem was intact. Each May, a festival is held in Fruita to celebrate the town's most famous fowl.)

The Desert RATS Trail Running Festival unfolds in mid-April, when the high desert is generally sunny but temperatures are well below their searing summer highs. Festivities begin on Friday night, with a pasta dinner in Grand Junction to prepare the longer-distance contestants for their sojourn on Saturday. Endurance runners have two options—a marathon or a 50K. (Marathon runners do a single long loop, while the 50K competitors do an additional 4.6-mile loop.) The route has a fairly gentle start on a rolling dirt road before climbing to the day's first single track. Here, you'll be treated to some broad vistas before a steep descent. Not long after, you'll reach Moore Fun and Mary's Loop—wide, fast, and flat. On the latter part of Mary's Loop the terrain becomes more technical, but this is balanced by stunning views of the mighty Colorado River. "The Moore Fun Trail is one of my favorite sections," Reid continued. "It's really rugged, but I love the beautiful overlook of the river and three layers of trail below you." With a little luck, you might spy golden eagles floating above the river or bighorn sheep clinging to the canyon walls.

After Moore Fun, you'll climb a little more than a mile to a point that has 360-degree views of both the trails below and the distant Book Cliffs. After another dip and climb you'll reach Pizza Overlook. From here, the trail follows a rim line in and out of a series of canyons. "It's a consistently picturesque course," Reid added, "but I think many find this portion the most scenic." From here, you'll come to the Crossroads Trail, which takes you to the last leg of the run, on the Troy Built Trail. A section of the course here hugs the overlook a bit close for some people's tastes, but then a steep descent leads you back onto the road. The finish line is not far ahead. (On Sunday, the 10K and half marathon are run on portions of these same trails.)

"Though the sport of running a race like the Desert RATS is intense, I'm always surprised at how friendly everyone is—even those who are looking to win. We try to keep this spirit going in our races. Everyone here is doing something amazing, and I feel we need to treat them that way.

"I'm a back-of-the-pack runner myself. At some events, no one is around when someone like me comes in. We reward those who come in quickly, but participants are also around for those who come in last." Top finishers, incidentally, receive a fitting prize—a cowbell bearing the race logo. "There's a lot of grazing land in the Fruita region," Reid explained, "so the cowbell seemed a fitting icon for the race. It also comes in handy at the finish line. Those who've already gotten their cowbell use it to cheer the runners in.

"At the after-party in Grand Junction, you can imagine how often people are playing the 'More Cowbell' clip from the *Saturday Night Live* episode."

REID DELMAN relocated to Boulder, Colorado, in 1994. When he and his wife, Michele, learned they would be having twins, they decided it was a perfect time for Reid to leave his job as a high school teacher and wrestling coach to be at home with the babies and start the business they'd always wanted—Gemini Adventures, which orchestrates the Desert RATS Trail Running Festival in addition to other events. Reid wrestled for Ohio State and recently competed in mixed martial arts cagefighting. He has completed many hundred-mile and fifty-mile running races and loves to make his own adventures—which is how he finds many of the racecourses currently offered by Gemini Adventures. He has also competed in adventure races, including the Eco-Challenge, mountain bike races, and Ironman Triathlons.

If You Go

▶ **Getting There:** The nearest airport is in Grand Junction, which is served by a number of airlines, including American (800-433-7300; aa.com) and United (800-864-8331; united.com).
▶ **Best Time to Visit:** The Desert RATS Trail Running Festival is held in mid-April.
▶ **Race Information:** The festival is operated by Gemini Adventures (303-249-1112; geminiadventures.com/running-events-2/festival); information about the race, including registration materials, can be found on the Gemini Adventures website.
▶ **Accommodations:** The Grand Junction Visitor & Convention Bureau (970-244-1480; visitgrandjunction.com) highlights area lodging options. Gemini Adventures designates a host hotel each year.

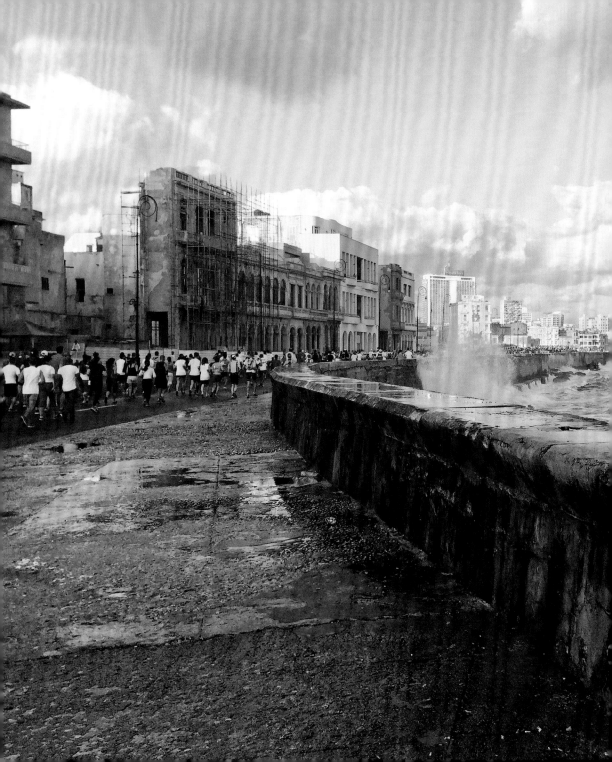

MARABANA

RECOMMENDED BY **Karen Hoch**

No running destination may have more mystique than Cuba. For runners like Karen Hoch, that's a big part of Havana's appeal.

"First, as an American you need to secure a 'highly sought after' visa in order to travel to Cuba, so there's a forbidden fruit appeal and a sense of special privilege—as someone participating in a sporting event, you can go when others may have more obstacles trying to travel there. There's also the allure of a lush, Caribbean island. Though the government is still in control of many aspects of Cuban life, there's so much activity and vibrancy. It draws you in. For me, the people make a place, and I really appreciate the Cuban people. Though they don't have much in a material sense, they seem happy and are very welcoming. I'm very visually oriented, and the colors of Havana are riveting, whether it's the buildings, the cars, or the greenery and flowers."

Much has been written about the status of Cuba as a country at a crossroads. At times, facets of the city of Old Havana seem to contradict one another. Grand colonial facades slowly crumble in the shadow of recently constructed (or renovated) five-star hotels. Street vendors hawk sundry biographies of Che Guevara under the eye of police while men and women furtively solicit passersby to visit their *paladares* (private in-home restaurants) as the ubiquitous 1950s American land yachts belch diesel fumes into the perpetually humid air. Though many of the original members of the Buena Vista Social Club have passed on, the strains of "Guantanamera" still float above the public squares . . . and still inspire romance. With Fidel Castro's passing and the rekindling of diplomatic relations with the United States, changes are likely to accelerate. Many travel insiders feel that the time to experience Cuba is as soon as possible . . . lest Havana turn into a giant theme park!

OPPOSITE:
Runners will feel the ocean's salty spray along the famed Malecón during Cuba's Marabana.

For runners seeking a good excuse to visit Cuba, there's the Marabana—a fusion of marathon and *Habana*. The route is a loop, which starts in front of the *Capitolio* at the edge of Old Havana, then makes its way along the Malecón, Havana's famed esplanade along Havana Harbor, before winding through a host of neighborhoods and circling back to the start. A marathon is two loops of this course; a great majority of runners—nearly 90 percent, in fact—opt for the half, 10K, or 5K alternatives. "In the years that I've led trips to the Marabana, I've found that a lot of people will sign up for the marathon," Karen continued, "but as we get closer to the event, they switch to the half marathon. I think they become a little less focused on the race itself and more on enjoying their short time in Cuba. That being said, we certainly have more advanced and focused runners who do the trip. One of our runners, a woman named Inez-Anne [Haagen] from the Netherlands, came in second place in the women's marathon division." (Karen pointed out that if you're planning to go the distance, you should be sure to bring powdered electrolytes and any other nutritional supplements you might desire, as you won't find them for sale in local markets. Nor will you find Gatorade along the course, though there's ample water.)

Initiated in 1987, the Marabana is Cuba's largest road race; in 2016, there were about 3,600 participants. "An appeal of the event is its modest size," Karen added. "They don't have corrals or waves. Everyone starts together, whichever distance you're going. It's very relaxed at the start; there's none of the tension you feel at some races—though focused runners who want a good time can position themselves accordingly. There are many international runners [more than 1,500 from sixty-four countries in 2016] in the field, and many sport their countries' colors or flags on their attire. Mingling with runners from Cuba and so many different places makes for a fun start. The joviality is complemented by live music."

For many runners, the early section of the course along the Malecón is a favorite. "The waves are sometimes crashing over the seawall," Karen described, "and many will stop to take pictures of runners getting splashed. You pass the US embassy, which is moving, given our history. Most of the runners are together at this time, so that sense of joyousness continues. Your adrenaline is going; before you even realize, you've run miles. When you turn off the Malecón, you come into neighborhoods that you might not encounter on a bus tour of Havana. This is an aspect of running in a city that I especially love—the chance to see more of daily life and how people live. On foot, you get a better sense of the place. As you make your way back toward Old Havana, you also see some of the more famous sites like Revolution Square and the national sports stadium. The finish is also special. It's downhill, which is always nice—and you can see the capitol building in the distance. While there's some support from Havanans along the route, there are tons of people cheering at the finish . . . and, of course, there's more music. I have run many races around the world, and seldom do I grab fellow runners' hands at the finish line, but I have each time in Havana. Somehow, this race captures the spirit of the Cuban people."

Sports are important to Cubans, and this extends to running. But a lack of proper gear is a challenge. "Some people at the Marabana are running barefoot or in sneakers like Converse with no support at all," Karen said. "Others might have running shoes so ancient that their toes are hanging out. We tell all of our guests to be prepared to give up their sneakers at the end of the race, as local people really need them. We encourage people to bring extras to give away; it's another way to feel good at the race's end."

When the running is done, Marathon Tours guests have the chance to take in a number of Havana's rich cultural attractions. Karen shared a few of her favorites. "I have enjoyed watching and trying salsa dancing. There are several places where you can find fabulous music and a great environment to try what comes so easy to the locals. Visiting Ernest Hemingway's house is another must. After being in the city for a few days, it's very peaceful, as the property is on a hill outside of town. Seeing the big pool and his old boat (*Pilar*), you can't help but imagine his life there."

KAREN HOCH has nearly twenty years of experience in travel logistics, conference planning, and marketing. She has completed nine marathons, including Boston's, and many half marathons. She is a certified running coach with the Road Runners Club of America and a Certified Meeting Professional (CMP). She earned her MS in marketing communications from the University of Kansas and BS in economics and finance from Bentley University. In addition to working on Marathon Tours & Travel marketing efforts, Karen manages the Italy Coast to Coast Relay and the company's programs in Big Sur, Cuba, Kenya, Madagascar, and New York. She recently returned from Jerusalem, which Marathon Tours & Travel is excited to add to their 2018 race calendar!

15

DESTINATION

If You Go

▶ **Getting There:** As of this writing, it's still technically illegal to travel to Cuba, though there are a number of exceptions . . . like athletic competitions. If you wish to go it alone, you'll want to start by visiting the Cuban embassy website (www.cubadiplomatica.cu) . . . though many will find it easier to arrange all travel through an outfitter like Marathon Tours (617-242-7845; marathontours.com).

▶ **Best Time to Visit:** The Marabana is generally held in November, when Havana is a bit cooler . . . but it's still best to plan on more heat and humidity than you'd encounter on most courses.

▶ **Race Information:** You can find details about the Marabana at mapoma.es/marabana.

▶ **Accommodations:** Karen recommends several downtown hotels, an easy walk to the race's start/finish, including Parque Central (hotelparquecentral-cuba.com) and Hotel Saratoga (hotel-saratoga.com); if you travel with Marathon Tours, they'll arrange all lodging and tours.

DESTINATION 15

MARINE CORPS MARATHON

RECOMMENDED BY **Rick Nealis**

Since its inception, the Marine Corps Marathon (MCM) has been called "the people's marathon." Some may see this as a catchy slogan, but for Rick Nealis, it pretty much sums up the spirit of the race. "When the US Marine Corps decided to assemble the first race in 1976, it was to showcase the Corps' organizational skills and to honor the nation's bicentennial. But we also wanted to keep the event focused on each and every runner. This wasn't going to be a New York, Chicago, or Boston Marathon, where the elite athletes get a lot of the attention. There wasn't going to be a purse for the winners. When you look at a lot of other big races, the courses are designed to focus on speed, with more straight lines. The Marine Corps Marathon has lots of turns. We want to show runners as many of Washington, DC's monuments and statues as possible. I ran my first marathon here in 1981, and I wasn't alone. More than 40 percent of our runners are first-time marathoners. The marines work hard to create a supportive environment.

"The race also is inspired by patriotism, and likewise inspires patriotism. It begins with the name. Most marathons are named for cities. The Marine Corps Marathon attracts attention to the marines and other armed forces members who are putting themselves in harm's way to protect the country. I think this is especially significant at this time, when America has been at war for fourteen years. In 2001, after the 9/11 attacks, the Marine Corps was the first major marathon held. We wanted to help rally the nation in a positive way."

The Marine Corps Marathon progenitor was a retired colonel named Jim Fowler. In addition to the goals Rick described above, Colonel Fowler was hoping to help boost the popularity of the military in light of the Vietnam War, and to embrace the enthusiasm for distance running that was sweeping across America at the time. The race could be

16

DESTINATION

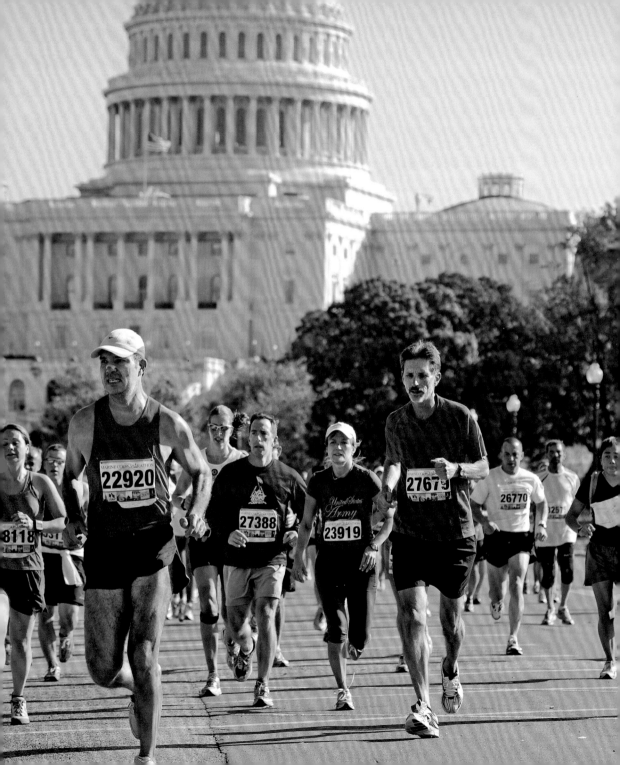

a soft recruiting tool and also a convenient way for running enthusiast marines to qualify for the Boston Marathon. With the help of a superior, General Michael Ryan, the first Marine Corps Reserve Marathon was run in November of 1976, with 1,018 participants—at the time the largest inaugural participation for a new marathon. For 1977, Colonel Fowler was able to enlist the further support of the chief of police for DC and bring the route past the district's more iconic sights—the route the marathon takes today. By 1978, the "Reserve" was dropped, and the race became the domain of the active duty Marine Corps.

The starting line for the MCM says a great deal about the event's symbolic significance. "We start at Arlington National Cemetery, in view of the Pentagon," Rick continued. "You're next to hallowed ground. As you're getting ready to run and glance over at Arlington, you can't help but think about what you're doing relative to the people resting in the cemetery, who've made the ultimate sacrifice. After four miles, you come into Georgetown on the DC side of the race, one of the city's oldest neighborhoods. The crowds are thick, and they energize you. Another great moment comes when you reach the National Mall and run past all its landmarks—older ones like the Lincoln Memorial and Washington Monument, and newer ones like the National Museum of African American History and Culture. When you cross the Fourteenth Street Bridge back into Virginia, you see the Pentagon again. Many of our runners are millennials, and half their life has been post 9/11, when we've been at war. Again, you can't help but reflect on our servicemen and women."

The success of Frank Shorter in the 1972 Olympics and Jim Fixx's bestselling 1977 title, *The Complete Book of Running*, did wonders to launch long-distance running into the mainstream. One of the next great boosts for the sport came in 1994, when Oprah Winfrey decided to run a marathon to commemorate her fortieth birthday . . . and chose the MCM. "I had heard that Oprah was planning to run the Chicago Marathon," Rick recalled. "That made sense, as she's from Chicago. But I thought it was worthwhile to reach out to her about the MCM. As a celebrity, she had so many distractions and security issues. The gist of the short letter I sent along to Harpo Productions [Winfrey's production company] was, 'You're a first-timer; you should be able to focus on running. Come run with the marines, and we'll protect you so you can focus!' This was in the early spring. In June, someone from her security team reached out. By July, we knew she was coming to Washington. She competed that October, and her time—

OPPOSITE:
The Marine Corps Marathon, known as "the people's marathon," takes runners past many of Washington, DC's landmarks.

DESTINATION **16**

4:29:15—became a rallying cry. People wanted to beat her time. After Oprah ran, we had record numbers of women registering to run. Running a marathon had been on her bucket list, like it is for many, and she checked it off. The MCM is all about dreams. You don't have to be superfast to realize your dream. We're always there to take care of the last runner."

Finishing any marathon is an exhilarating experience. But the finish at the Marine Corps Marathon is something even the most seasoned marathoners are unlikely to forget. "You've gone twenty-six miles, and all of a sudden, the last three hundred yards are uphill," Rick described. "It feels like a mountain. You want to walk. But either side of the road is filled with marines cheering you on, and the energy is incredible. When you reach the top, you see the Marine Corps War Memorial—the statue of the six marines raising the US flag on top of Mount Suribachi during the battle of Iwo Jima. It pulls you like a magnet. When you cross the finish line, a US marine places a finishing medal around your neck and says, 'Good job, sir' or 'Good job, ma'am.' This reflects the respect the marines have for finishers. We have thousands of civilian volunteers for the event, but only a current duty marine can present your medal. These days, many people may not have ever seen a US marine in person. This is a chance to be up close and personal with a marine—have a discussion, perhaps even share a hug."

It's a magical moment.

RICK NEALIS was commissioned in the US Marine Corps in 1975, after graduating from Villanova University. His twenty-year military career includes deployments aboard the USS *Tarawa*, USS *Okinawa*, and the USS *Tripoli*, as part of the amphibious ready group during the Iranian hostage rescue attempt. While in the US Marine Corps, Rick furthered his education, earning an MBA in management from Golden State University and an MS in human organizational services from Villanova. He joined the MCM staff in 1993. In 1994, he organized Oprah Winfrey's participation in the MCM. Following retirement from the Marine Corps, Rick served as the Olympic torch deputy caravan coordinator for the Centennial Olympic Games in Atlanta. He carried the Olympic torch during the longest leg of the relay occurring in Young Harris, Georgia, on July 16, 1996. On December 19, 2001, he again carried the Olympic torch in Uniontown, Pennsylvania. In 2002, Rick served as a member of the security team for the Olympic Torch Relay at the Olympic Games in Salt Lake City. In 2009, Rick was inducted into the Running USA

Hall of Champions, and in 2010, he was named Race Director of the Year by Road Race Management and MarathonFoto. Rick has completed five marathons (including three MCMs) and boasts a PR of 3:09:50, obtained at the 1983 MCM.

If You Go

▶ **Getting There:** Washington, DC, is served by most major carriers.
▶ **Best Time to Visit:** The Marine Corps Marathon is held in late October.
▶ **Race Information:** Contact the MCM (800-RUN-USMC; marinemarathon.com) for everything you need to know about the event, including the race's lottery registration.
▶ **Accommodations:** The MCM lists a number of partner hotels on its website. Destination DC (800-422-8644; washington.org) lists other lodging options around the US capital.

16

DESTINATION

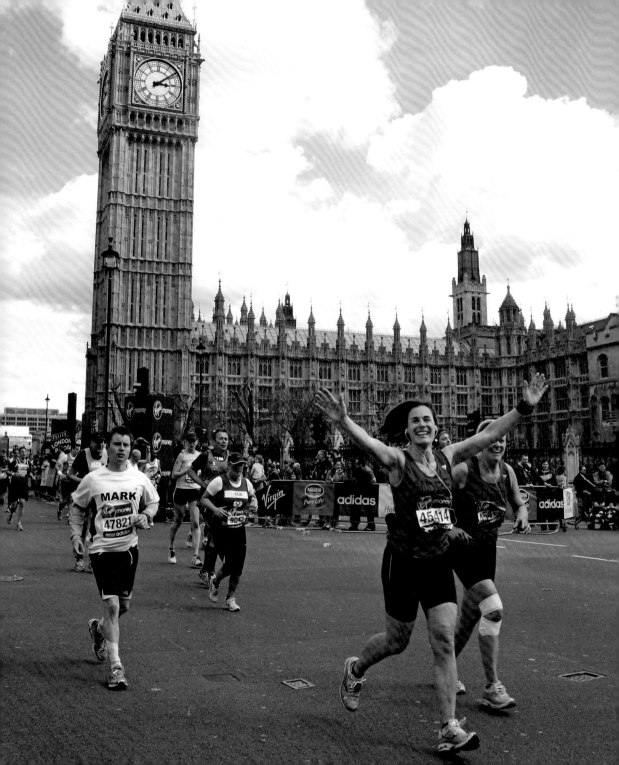

LONDON MARATHON

RECOMMENDED BY **David Bedford**

Former ten thousand meters world record holder David Bedford did not take the standard approach to running his first London Marathon. "At the time—1981—I had finished my serious running career, though I was certainly aware that the event was taking place," he recalled. "I owned a nightclub in Luton (just north of London) at the time, and one of the punters in the club got me into a bet that I couldn't run the marathon the next day. I'd had a few beers at the time, and I took his bet . . . and changed from beer to piña coladas. I was a bit worse for wear, but when the race started the next morning at nine o'clock, I was there. I finished in three hours and forty-five minutes—not my best time—but to be honest, I was delighted to have finished. Though I won the bet, I was never paid." The payment, at least from a karmic perspective, came a bit later: In the year 2000, David was named race director.

The London Marathon (now Virgin Money London Marathon) was conceived by two members of the Ranelagh Harriers, John Disley and Chris Brasher. The group regularly met at a pub called the Dysart Arms, and one night over pints of bitters, there was talk of the New York Marathon, which several club members had run in 1978. Disley and Brasher decided to journey across the pond to try it for themselves in 1979. Upon finishing, they couldn't help but imagine the great city of London one day hosting a marathon to rival the race of the young upstart in America. The idea of such a large-scale run posed a number of challenges, not least of which was the closing of twenty-six miles of road and several bridges (including the iconic Tower Bridge). But Disley and Brasher were able to secure both police approval for the route and a sponsor (Gillette—though since 2008 the sponsor has been Virgin Money), as the city fathers refused to underwrite the event. The inaugural race in March of 1981 saw 7,747 runners leave the starting line, and 6,255

OPPOSITE:
London
Marathon
participants
experience some
two thousand
years of history
in 26.2 miles.

DESTINATION

17

87

crossed the finish. The following year, there were ninety thousand applications from would-be entrants, and more than eighteen thousand runners participated.

A race worthy of the city had been born.

"When Chris and John first assembled the event, they had two challenges," David continued. "To help ensure that it could grow into a major event, they had to make the course as fast as possible while passing as many iconic landmarks as possible. While the course has many twists and turns and is not quite as fast as Berlin, London has had its share of world records. Finding a large open area for the start was critical, and Blackheath (in southeast London) fit the bill. From there, the hope was to follow the River Thames as much as possible. In those early days, London was being massively rebuilt, so there were constant changes to the course to accommodate that—though the start and finish [near Buckingham Palace] have remained constant. In considering any alterations, the goal of keeping a fast course was a driving factor." After leaving Blackheath, runners reach *Cutty Sark* (the famed clipper ship, not the scotch) in Greenwich after roughly six miles. You'll cross the meridian line (as in Greenwich Mean Time) and then cross the River Thames at Tower Bridge, London's most popular tourist site. "From here, the route then turns into the East End," David explained. "This was once a dull, rather desolate part of the city, but now it's been rebuilt with Canary Wharf and London's new financial center. Then it comes back toward the center of London, past many iconic landmarks—the London Eye [also known as the Millennium Wheel], the Houses of Parliament, and Big Ben, to end on the Mall in front of Buckingham Palace. Over 26.2 miles, runners experience two thousand years of London history."

The London Marathon attracts more than six hundred thousand spectators, making it perhaps the city's greatest outdoor celebration. "It's one of the longest street parties in the world," David added. "There are seventy-five bands spread along the route, and many of the pubs that are passed have their best day of the year. Overall, it's a very festive atmosphere. I think the runners have as much fun looking at the spectators as they do taking in the sights."

One of David's most abiding memories of the London Marathon—a memory likely shared by many around the world—is Michael Watson's determined completion of the course in 2003. Watson was a professional boxer until he received a near fatal blow from Chris Eubank as the two competed for the World Boxing Organization super middle-weight title on a fateful night in 1991 that left him with severe brain injuries. After forty days in a coma and six brain operations, he seemed to have little hope of recovery. But within a year his speech returned, then he was able to use a wheelchair, and he eventually regained the ability to walk. In 2003, in an effort to raise funds for the Brain & Spine Foundation, he set out to show the world he was still a fighter, walking two hours each morning and afternoon for six days until he crossed the finish line with a time of six days, two hours, twenty-seven minutes, and seventeen seconds. As he finished, Chris Eubank, who'd become a close friend, was at his side.

"There are people who make it difficult for themselves to finish the marathon," David mused, "pushing things along or dressing up. The spirit of the London Marathon was never shown more powerfully than when Michael completed it, without making it any harder than life had already made it for him. It's here that the true spirit of the marathon resides."

DAVID BEDFORD is a former race director of the London Marathon and chairman of the IAAF Road Running Commission, and was once a world record holder in the ten thousand meters. In addition to his many running achievements, both as a competitor and an administrator, David has been a teacher and a nightclub owner. He also held British records in the three-thousand-meter steeplechase and five thousand meters, and competed in the 1972 Olympics. In 2014, David was appointed Officer of the Order of the British Empire in recognition of his services to athletics and charitable fund-raising.

If You Go

▶ **Getting There:** London is served by most international carriers.
▶ **Best Time to Visit:** The Virgin Money London Marathon is generally held on the fourth Sunday in April.
▶ **Race Information:** You can review event details and complete an entry form at the marathon's website (virginmoneylondonmarathon.com).
▶ **Accommodations:** Lodging packages at partner hotels are highlighted at the marathon's website. Visit London (visitlondon.com) lists a host of other lodging options.

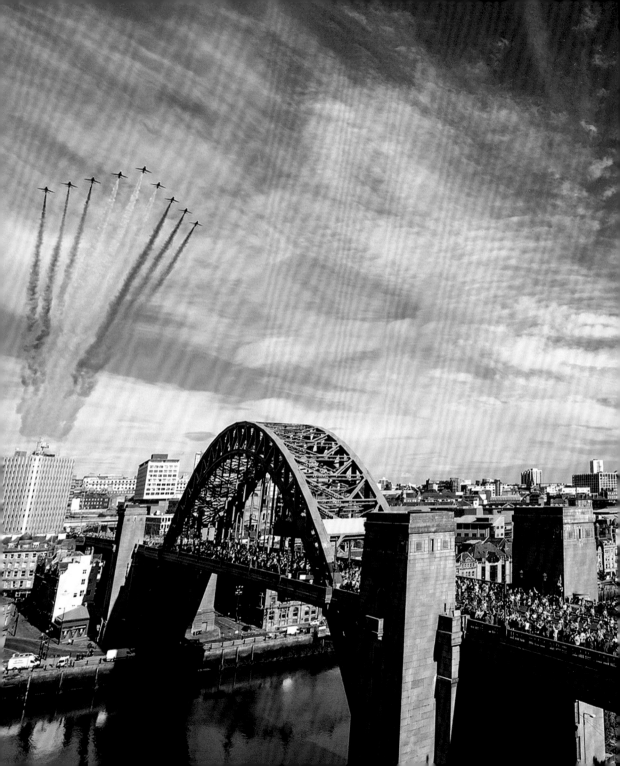

GREAT NORTH RUN

RECOMMENDED BY **John Caine**

In the late 1970s, the River Tyne was so polluted it more resembled a large sewage ditch than a river, and the northeast England city it flowed through—Newcastle—was rapidly becoming a poster child for postindustrial blight. Forty years later, the River Tyne is one of the United Kingdom's most healthy and prolific Atlantic salmon rivers, and Newcastle has been recognized as one of the best cities in the United Kingdom, with attractions like the tilting Gateshead Millennium Bridge, Baltic Centre for Contemporary Art, and the stunning Sage Gateshead concert hall. What changed? For one thing, the Great North Run was launched. "I can't say that the Great North was responsible for the economic revitalization of Newcastle and Tyneside," John Caine offered, "but it boosted the confidence of our citizens and demonstrated the personality of the region to the rest of Great Britain. It showed that the Northeast was a good place." Today, the Simplyhealth Great North Run—a half marathon—attracts more than fifty-seven thousand entrants and some forty-two thousand finishers, making it the largest half marathon in the world.

Some may not think of Greater Newcastle as a hotbed of competitive running, yet this is a misperception. "Tyneside has a rich history of running and rowing going back to the 1840s and '50s," John continued. "During Victorian times, match running was hugely popular. The races—five or ten miles or twenty-four hours—would draw enormous crowds, in part because there was gambling associated with the races. This culture died out with the rise of the modern Olympics and the growth of amateur sport. But the running clubs endured. I met Brendan Foster at such a club, the Gateshead Harriers, in 1964 as juniors. Brendan, of course, went on to many great achievements, including several world records and an Olympic bronze medal in the ten thousand meters in 1976. Toward the end of his professional career in the winter of 1979 and 1980, Brendan was training

OPPOSITE:
Runners crossing
the Tyne Bridge
at the outset of
the Great North
Run as the Red
Arrows fly above.

DESTINATION

18

in New Zealand. He and Dave Moorcroft [another British Olympic runner] happened to participate in a fun run in Auckland called Round the Bays. The notion of such runs didn't really exist in Europe at the time, and Brendan was taken with the idea. He told Dave, 'When I get home, I'm going to organize one of these.'

"Brendan was good to his word. That December, after the Moscow Olympics, he gathered me and three other friends from the Gateshead Harriers to plan a massive run. We divided up responsibilities: I was to find the route and be race director, Dave Roberts would manage the start, Max Coleby the route and medical support, John Trainor the finish, and Brendan would organize sponsors and work with the media. The most iconic landmark in Newcastle is the Tyne Bridge, which was built by the same company that later built the famed bridge in Sydney. This had to be part of the route, but trying to start from this point was making it difficult to get the proper distances. We knew we wanted to end at the coast, and a half marathon seemed right. When I began working backward, the route came together after a few weeks of jiggering. We were able to get permission from the chief of police and the city fathers for the three boroughs the proposed route would pass through. Then we just needed a name. The road that goes over the Tyne Bridge used to be called the Great North Road; it went from London to Edinburgh. It was a name that people could identify instantly, so we grabbed it."

Thanks to Brendan's heroic reputation and the novelty of the idea, the inaugural Great North Run received tremendous coverage on both local television and in the print media. That June of 1981, it had more than 12,000 entrants and 10,200 finishers, making it the United Kingdom's biggest running event. "Unbeknownst to us, at the same time we were hatching the Great North, Chris Brasher and John Disley were pulling together the first London Marathon, which debuted in April of that year," John added. "We still have the edge on them in terms of entry numbers." In 2015, the millionth runner completed the Great North. The lucky lady received a number of prizes, including a trip to New Zealand to participate in Round the Bays.

The Great North Run starts with a bang. "We always have a celebrity starter, someone with a connection to Tyneside," John described. (Past starters have included Sting, Mark Knopfler, Frank Williams [Formula One team boss], and various UK Olympic champions.) "The Red Arrows [the Royal Air Force equivalent of the Blue Angels] fly over the starting grid, then cruise just above the Tyne Bridge blasting out red, white, and blue trailer smoke. Runners cross the Tyne Bridge after a mile or so—the bridge is five or six deep with spectators. At mile three, you pass Gateshead Stadium, where Brendan broke the three thousand meters world record in 1974. Several miles in the countryside follow before runners come into the town of South Shields. At mile 11.5, you have a slight climb. When you crest the hill, there's an expansive view of the North Sea. You drop 250 meters onto the coast road. For the last mile, the sea is on your right and crowds on the left. There are more than one hundred thousand people between runners and spectators at the finish, which is right next to the estuary. The Red Arrows return and do a full aerobatic display."

The success of the Great North spawned new interest in running among the north country's youngsters. Brendan and his cohorts responded with a 5K, a 3K, and a mini-run. In 2011, a city center track meet was established during the Great North weekend, with US, UK, European, and Commonwealth teams competing. (There's an adjacent pasta party for fourteen-thousand-plus!) And thanks to the demand created by the success of the Great North, the Great Run Company now operates fun runs all over the United Kingdom.

The positive energy that the Great North has brought to once downtrodden Newcastle has spread much further afield. "A newly appointed British ambassador to Ethiopia, Myles Wickstead, wanted to make a positive British impression on the country," John shared. "At the time, 2000, Ethiopia was well known for famine, civil war, etc. The only positive thing outsiders associated with the country was its fantastic runners. Wickstead thought, 'Can't we do something with this?' A young woman in his office said, 'My mom knows Brendan Foster, who organized the Great North Run.' Soon a meeting was arranged. I traveled to Addis Ababa, met with the mayor, chief of police, and media. We instigated the idea of involving the great Ethiopian champion Haile Gebrselassie in the event, and created the Great Ethiopian Run, a 10K in Addis Ababa. The first race had ten thousand entrants. In 2016, it had forty thousand entrants. It's now completely managed by Ethiopian folks and is unlike any running event in the world."

JOHN CAINE is now retired but was the race director of the Great North Run for twenty years. Old injuries curtail his running, so he hikes, goes fishing, does woodwork, and drinks beer, as well as serves on the board of the Great Run Company.

DESTINATION 18

If You Go

▶ **Getting There:** Newcastle is served by a number of carriers, including British Airways (800-247-9297; britishairways.com) and Ryanair (+44 8712460002; ryanair.com).

▶ **Best Time to Visit:** The Great North Run is generally held on the second Sunday in September.

▶ **Race Information:** You'll find everything you need to know about the Great North Run at greatrun.org.

▶ **Accommodations:** Nirvana Europe (nirvanaeurope.com), the event's official travel partner, can help you with a range of lodging options. Entries are filled by January, so plan early.

18

DESTINATION

EVERGLADES ULTRAS

RECOMMENDED BY **Bob Becker**

"I started producing races in 2008," Bob began, "including the Keys 100, an ultra that goes from Key Largo to Key West. I enjoyed the experience and wanted to stay at it. One of the Keys 100 participants from New York had a good friend in Naples who was a big trail runner. When the guy in Naples heard about the Keys event, he called me and said he had done some running in a place called the Fakahatchee Strand Preserve State Park, and he thought it could make a great venue for an event."

The Fakahatchee Strand Preserve State Park rests roughly twenty-five miles east of Naples and is Florida's largest—and perhaps least well known—state park. Its eighty-five thousand acres make up the lion's share of the Fakahatchee Strand, a linear swamp forest that's home to one of the largest concentrations of native orchids in North America, as well as many of Florida's rare and endangered animals. These include the Florida panther and Florida black bear, as well as the less endangered but no less impressive alligator. "It's quite a varied environment," Bob continued. "Part of it is jungle, part of it is swamp, the extremely lush terrain people expect when they think of this region. But there are also open prairie lands and thickly wooded areas. A change of elevation of a few feet makes a major difference. The varied environment makes it a beautiful place to run."

Bob continued to explain the evolution of the Everglades Ultras, which offers a fifty-mile race, a 50K race, and a 25K race. "I contacted the park manager and explained how I organized these long races. She thought I was nuts. The more I talked, though, the more she realized it could make sense. Fakahatchee is underutilized, and a race would help promote the park. It would also provide some low-cost maintenance. To create a fifty-mile trail run, many miles of trail would have to be cleared. The park only has a staff of four. We'd bring in volunteers to help open up the trails, which could be used by visitors to bike, hike, and run. It would also facilitate passage to areas that were generally inaccessible for fire control and other maintenance needs. The park gets a great deal of support from the Friends of Fakahatchee, a volunteer organization. They were understandably skittish about several hundred people coming out, thinking they might damage sensitive areas or leave trash. They eventually bought into the notion. I think they came to understand that trail runners were very respectful of the environment."

It would've been very difficult to carve any kind of trail through the Fakahatchee—let alone running trails—without the legacy of the area's cypress forests. "The cypress trees were heavily logged in the forties and fifties," Bob explained, "but considering that cypresses grow in swamps, the loggers needed a way to get them out. They would dig ditches and put the dirt in the center, creating a raised area above the swamp. Then they'd level it off and put in a narrow-gauge railroad. These tram roads are the basis of the trail system that we helped clear." Bob and a team of volunteers have thus far cleared away more than seventy miles of trail.

The course of the Everglades Ultras varies a bit each year, depending on how much water is present. "We do the race in February, as that's typically the driest month in the Everglades; it's a bit cooler and there are fewer mosquitoes," Bob said. "But occasionally— like in 2015—there was so much water many sections were inaccessible." One constant is that the fifty-mile runners begin in the dark. (The 50K and 25K runners begin later, each staggered by 1.5 hours.) "We stress safety," Bob continued. "All runners must have a head lamp. The first 6.25 miles are on a dirt road, so for all but the fastest runners, it's starting to get light by the time they reach the tram roads. It's a memorable start in the dark, with the bellowing calls of alligators and bullfrogs and scattering birds. One of the run's special moments comes a few miles up the first tram road, where there's a cabin— one of a few private landholdings within the park. The cabin, which we call the Fakahatchee Hilton, is on a huge alligator pond. Many runners will stop here to watch gators; there might be twenty-five or thirty looking up at you from the pond.

"It's not uncommon to see other animals on the trails. Most days, there aren't many people on the trail. When you have two-hundred-plus runners coming through, they are scattering around. I've seen a panther and black bear out there. But we do have rangers patrolling on the active trails to make sure there are no alligators on the tram."

Though conditions in February are preferable to the rest of the year, it's still warm and humid. Bob offered some tips for runners to stay comfortable. "Wear a hat to protect your head, ideally one with a neck drape. Wear a neck bandanna or a buff under your hat and take advantage of the ice available at aid stations along the way. Be sure to take in enough electrolytes and calories. We allow runners to utilize drop bags with food and changes of clothes at aid stations before the race begins. We try to provide as much support as possible to help runners manage the heat."

BOB BECKER has run the Boston Marathon, climbed Mount Kilimanjaro, and raced in the 150-mile Marathon des Sables stage race in the Sahara Desert in Morocco and the 167-mile Grand to Grand Ultra stage race in the southwestern United States . . . all since turning fifty-seven! In addition to completing the 120-mile TransRockies stage race in Colorado, he has two top-fifty finishes at the Badwater® 135, is the oldest person who has run a Badwater Double (in 2015 at age seventy), and has completed multiple 150-mile races. A radical prostate cancer survivor, Bob found a passion for creating, producing, and directing long-distance running events, and has introduced ultramarathon racing to thousands of athletes in South Florida and beyond, including the Keys 100 and the Everglades Ultras. Bob's ultramarathon events raise money to combat prostate and other cancers through the Cancer Foundation of the Florida Keys, and in support of the spectacular but underfunded Fakahatchee Strand Preserve State Park. His individual races have also raised money for the National MS Society. He's been featured in the *Miami Herald*, *Runner's World*, *Trail Runner*, *Running Times*, and *Masters Athlete*, among others.

If You Go

▶ **Getting There:** The Fakahatchee Strand Preserve State Park is located in Copeland, Florida, roughly 1.5 hours from Miami, which is served by most major carriers.
▶ **Best Time to Visit:** The Everglades Ultras is held in mid-February, the driest time of year in the Everglades.
▶ **Race Information:** The Everglades Ultras website (evergladesultras.com) details the event, including registration information. The race is limited to three hundred participants.
▶ **Accommodations:** The Ivey House (239-695-3299; iveyhouse.com) is the official lodging provider for the event. Other options are listed at evergladesultras.com.

19

DESTINATION

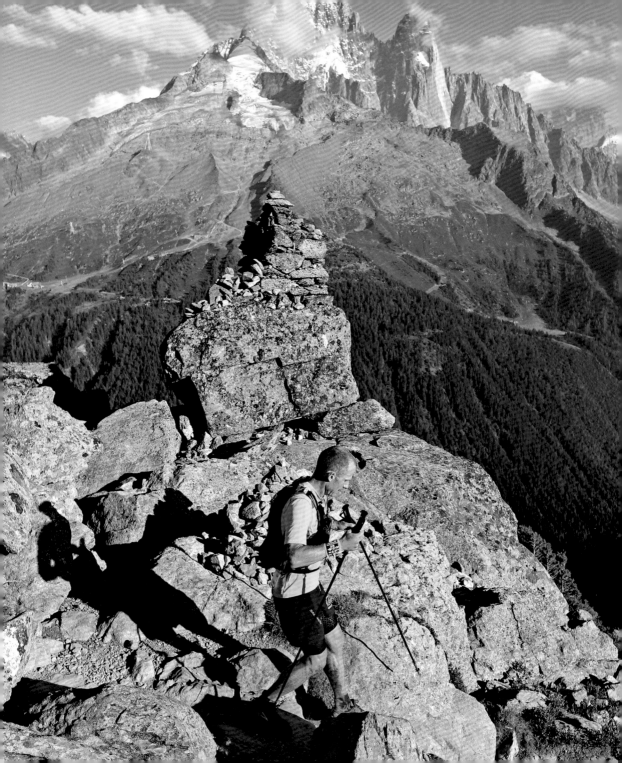

ULTRA-TRAIL DU MONT-BLANC

RECOMMENDED BY **Magdalena Lewy Boulet**

Magda Boulet set her sights on the Ultra-Trail du Mont-Blanc (UTMB)—the epic endurance race that circles the Mont Blanc massif, near the nexus of France, Italy, and Switzerland—after winning the Western States® Endurance Run in 2015. "For a driven personality like mine, I began to think, 'What's next? What's bigger?' I'd been watching the UTMB for a while, though this event hasn't received as much attention in the United States as a race like the Western States. I was blown away by the difficulty of the course, the challenge of it. It seemed bigger than something I could handle . . . especially given the logistics of trying to train for something like this when you live at sea level. But at the same time, it was attractive.

"In 2015, I did the CCC [Courmayeur–Champex–Chamonix], a 100K race that covers some parts of the UTMB course. I went with the goal of being a student, seeing if the UTMB would be a good fit. That race really won me over. Being in Chamonix and being part of something so grand was overwhelming. I wanted to be part of that energy."

Launched in 2001, the UTMB takes runners on a truly heroic trek, covering more than thirty-one thousand feet in elevation gain over 103 miles while touching three countries (Italy and Switzerland in addition to France). The race, which begins and ends in Chamonix, follows the famed Tour du Mont-Blanc trail—a route that's generally covered by hikers in seven to nine days. (The fastest UTMB finishers complete the course in a bit more than twenty hours under good conditions.) The highest point on the course is the Grand Col Ferret, which sits at 8,323 feet on the border with Switzerland. During the race's daylight hours—weather permitting—runners are treated to ever-shifting vistas of the Alps' tallest mountain (Mont Blanc sits at 15,774 feet). At times, your only company may be curious ibex, a species of wild goat that calls the Alps home.

OPPOSITE:
The UTMB
circles the Alps'
tallest mountain
and reaches
heights of more
than 8,300 feet.

20

DESTINATION

As the UTMB 2016 approached, Magda felt that she was ready. "I had a good taste of the course," she recalled. "And the CCC had been very manageable. It starts in the morning, lasts thirteen or fourteen hours, and is done in the evening. The UTMB is a different beast. You start in the evening, so for the first part of the race, you have to know how to race at night . . . and there's the potential you might go into another night. The beginning of the race is incredibly powerful. You and several thousand other runners are about to embark on a journey into the unknown. The race organizers do a wonderful job emphasizing how special your adventure will be. You get chills. Once the gun goes off, it's different. Mont Blanc is looking at you in downtown Chamonix. It feels very close, and the many unknowns ahead are almost overwhelming.

"My first night went pretty smoothly. But the next day it was extremely hot, and in the afternoon a big thunderstorm developed. I was on top of a mountain holding metal poles, with night approaching, and I was on my last big climb. It was pouring rain, there was lightning, and I was on a technical part of the course. Usually, this is not my strength. But when you're scared, you can become really good at something. I felt like I was running for my life. I learned a lot about myself."

This experience underscores an important part of preparation for the UTMB: an understanding of wilderness survival. "It's not enough to spend time training in the dark," Magda advised. "You need to spend time on mountain trails in the dark. You don't want that experience to be a first for you. You have to be ready for situations where you might be alone out there, even though there are three thousand other people on the course. You're running around a big mountain, and things can change. It's not just about being fit. It's about knowing how to deal with the elements."

A staggering distance. A punishing amount of climbing. Potential for dangerous, even life-threatening conditions. A more casual runner might ask, "Why?" Magda has certainly considered this question. "You sign up for more than the competition," she mused. "It's the experience. To finish a brutal ninety-minute climb and then be rewarded with this breathtaking view of one section of the mountain, and then watch the mountain become fogged ten minutes later. You live for those moments."

This celebration of experience, rather than competitive success, extends to the finish line at the UTMB. "You're beyond tired when you're finished," Magda said. "Part of you wants to lie down, though it's more comfortable to keep moving. And some of your friends are still out. When I ran the UTMB, I had a friend who didn't have as good a day.

I waited seven hours for him to come in. There's a lot of community around this race. Even in the middle of the night, people are waiting for their fellow runners."

MAGDALENA LEWY BOULET earned a spot on the US Olympic Team by finishing second in the women's marathon at the 2008 US Olympic Trials. She also won two team bronze medals as the captain of the US cross-country team at the World Cross Country Championships in 2010 and 2011. After a ten-year career running marathons on the road, Magda transitioned to running trail and ultra-distance events in 2013. In 2015, Magda won her hundred-mile debut at the prestigious Western States Endurance Run and was named North American Ultra-Runner of the Year. A native of Poland, she earned her bachelor's degree in human biodynamics from UC Berkeley in 1997 and a master's degree in exercise physiology from Cal State Hayward. In 2007, she returned to her alma mater as a coach for the Golden Bear cross-country program, where she coached cross-country and distance events for two years. Magda has been coached by Jack Daniels, PhD, a world-renowned authority on distance running, since 2001. She lives in Oakland, California, with her husband, Richie, one of the United States' best milers in the 1990s, and their son, Owen. Currently Magda leads innovation and product development at GU Energy Labs and enjoys training and competing in ultra-endurance trail races.

20

DESTINATION

If You Go

▶ **Getting There:** The nearest international airport is in Geneva, which is roughly 50 miles from Chamonix.

▶ **Best Time to Visit:** The UTMB is held in late August. The Tour du Mont-Blanc is generally free of snow from June through September, and there are huts along the way should you not wish to bite off all 103 miles at once.

▶ **Race Information:** Details about the UTMB and the other four endurance events held in Chamonix reside at utmbmontblanc.com.

▶ **Accommodations:** The Chamonix Tourist Office (+33 0450530024; chamonix.com) highlights lodging options in the region.

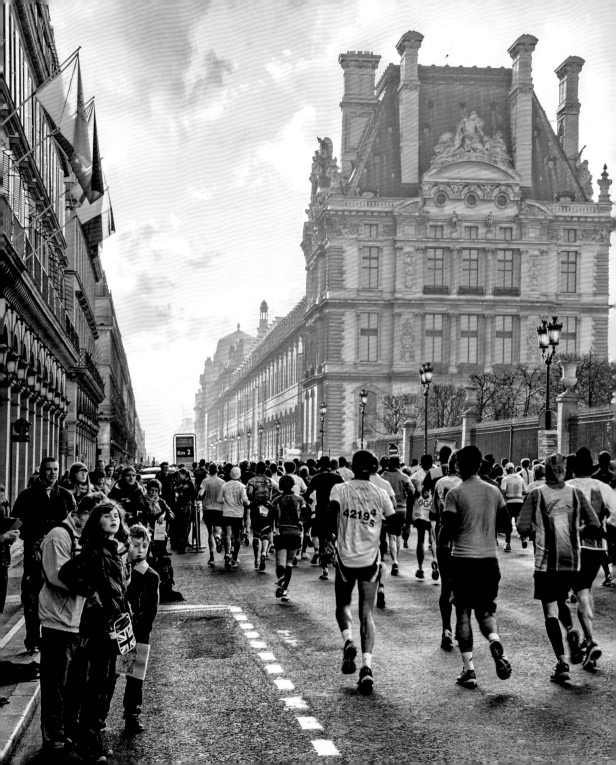

PARIS MARATHON

RECOMMENDED BY **Pascal Silvestre**

Ah, April in Paris! The perfume of freshly baked baguettes mixing with the first blossoms of spring. The sun climbing ever higher in the sky to better bathe the city in its special light. And on the second Sunday of the month, the thunder of nearly one hundred thousand sneakers pounding the pavement as runners from around the world compete in the Schneider Electric Paris Marathon.

"In the early nineties, I worked for several years in New York," Pascal Silvestre began. "I started running there, and I knew I one day wanted to run a marathon. My dream was to do the New York Marathon, but I returned to Paris to live. That was my first marathon; after that, I was hooked. I've now run the Paris Marathon twelve times, eleven times in a row. It's always a gift to be able to run through Paris, the most beautiful city in the world—or at least one of them. It's a special moment of the year to be able to be in Paris as spring arrives. There's a sense of rebirth in the air, and it's a great time to be running. We've been very lucky the last sixteen years. Once or twice we've had chilly, windy days, but most of the time we've had blue skies and perfect temperatures for running."

The very first Paris Marathon (known then as the Tour de Paris Marathon) was held in 1896, on the heels of the first modern Olympics. A distance of forty kilometers (24.85 miles) was selected, as this was the distance from the battlefields at Marathon to Athens. One hundred and ninety-one runners raced from Porte Maillot to Conflans-Sainte-Honorine. There was a hiatus of eighty years before the next marathon was held in Paris. This time around, the course was extended to the standard 42.195-kilometer (or 26.2-mile) length. Since the first modern Paris Marathon was run in 1976, the course has changed a number of times. These days, it's run completely on the Right Bank of the Seine and sees approximately fifty thousand runners.

OPPOSITE:
The modern Paris Marathon unfolds along the Right Bank of the Seine and sees nearly fifty thousand runners.

DESTINATION 21

103

Whether you're a lover of Paris and want an opportunity to commune with the City of Light or you're a newcomer hoping to experience the place you've heard so much about, the Paris Marathon will satisfy. Pascal went on to describe the course. "All the runners converge on the Champs-Elysées, where the race begins," he said. "You have the Arc de Triomphe [which honors soldiers who perished in the French Revolutionary and Napoleonic Wars] in front. The first two miles head downhill and bring you past the Place de la Concorde [one of the city's major squares]. You pass the Louvre and then the Place de la Bastille [where the infamous Bastille prison stood until it was dismantled during the revolution of 1789–90]. Here, you begin to pass through the markets. The smells of freshly baked bread, roasted chicken, and other foods are very tangible. You can't help but start thinking about what you'll treat yourself to after the race is done. Soon after, you enter a park, the Bois de Vincennes, which is Paris's largest park. After circling through the woods here, the route heads west along the river, back toward the center of the city. You pass Notre Dame, the Musée d'Orsay, the Eiffel Tower, and through another park, the Bois de Boulogne, before reaching the finish. This is my playground, where I train. But on the day of the race, it's that much more special."

Runners who feed off the energy of an enthusiastic crowd to push them past "the wall" may find the spectatorship in Paris a bit lacking. "In New York, when the marathon is happening, it's the main event of the day," Pascal opined. "In Paris, it's not a focal point. In fact, many Parisians may not know it's even happening." The low-key personality of the Paris Marathon extends to post-race festivities. "The French aren't into big pre- and post-race events," Pascal added. "Many finishers will join friends and go to a local restaurant. You won't see many runners wearing their medals. It's just not the French way. My group of running friends will usually select a bar to meet at after the race and enjoy a few beers." (The notion of French runners gathering for a few *beers* may seem foreign to some, but Paris has seen an explosion of craft brewers in the last ten years— not in the least because France is Europe's largest barley producer and the world's greatest exporter of malt.)

Given his dozen circuits of the Paris Marathon, Pascal has a passel of great memories of the run through the world's most beautiful city. "My first time, in 1996, I was shy and didn't know if I could finish. I didn't mention that I was participating to anyone; when I finished, I cried. After that, I was more organized in my training, and I ran the course nine times in under three hours. In 2011, I was asked to be a pacer—what an amazing day! I felt a huge responsibility, as the runners I was pacing had put so much energy into trying to break the three-hour mark. I'll never forget their hugs and handshakes after we finished. When you see people finishing, it's overwhelming—their fatigue, their emotion. For many, it's the experience of a lifetime. It's not only a marathon, but it's the *Paris Marathon*."

PASCAL SILVESTRE began running in 1994 when he quit smoking. He's gone on to run fifty-seven marathons, including New York City, Boston, Miami, Chicago, Marine Corps, San Francisco, Big Sur, Sedona, and Paris. Pascal created the website Runners (runners. fr), France's leading running site, and is also the author of *Marathon*, a collection of ten short stories that involve the marathon experience.

If You Go

▶ **Getting There:** Paris is served by most major carriers. Special travel packages from Air France (800-237-2747; airfrance.us) and KLM (866-434-0320; klm.com) are available for marathon participants.
▶ **Best Time to Visit:** The Schneider Electric Paris Marathon is generally held the second Sunday in April.
▶ **Race Information:** Entry forms and other information are available at www.schneider electricparismarathon.com.
▶ **Accommodations:** The French Tourist Office (francetourism.com) lists a broad assortment of lodging options around Paris.

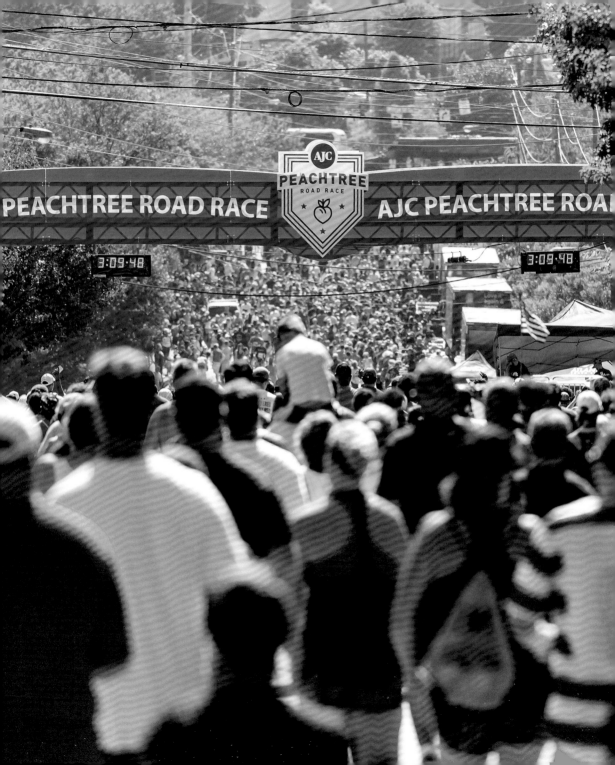

PEACHTREE ROAD RACE

RECOMMENDED BY **Amanda Kowaleski**

On July 4, 1970, a cross-country coach from Georgia State University named Tim Singleton assembled a group of 150 runners at an old Sears parking lot off Peachtree Road to do a race through the heart of Atlanta. The runners each put two dollars in a cigar box (to create a winner's purse) and took off. One hundred and ten finished in Central City Park. On July 4, 2016, some sixty thousand runners and walkers gathered around the starting line in Atlanta's Buckhead neighborhood to participate in what has grown to become America's largest running event—the Peachtree Road Race.

"I had always been fairly athletic, but I became a consistent runner once I moved to Atlanta," Amanda Kowaleski began. "I lived near Piedmont Park, so it was very easy. I first learned about the Peachtree when I was working for a television station in town, and I ended up field-producing the event. The Peachtree turned out to be the first organized race I ever ran. It was surreal, going from being a casual runner to running in the world's biggest 10K, especially as I had seen it from the other side. There was such excitement, as you have fifty-five thousand (at the time) people streaming in on MARTA [Atlanta's public transit system], all with their race numbers on, and the huge American flag hanging above the starting line. I travel on the roads the course takes all the time, but when the roads are shut down, you see Atlanta from a completely different perspective. It felt as though I'd never experienced the city until then."

The Peachtree Road Race course highlights the city that's come to be known as the shining capital of the New South, reflecting Atlanta's ever-climbing skyline as well as its ascendancy as a business and cultural powerhouse. Amanda described the route. "The race starts in Buckhead, one of the busiest neighborhoods in Atlanta. There are two big malls and many high-rises right by the start line. It has a big-city feeling, and it's an

OPPOSITE:
The Peachtree
Road Race is
held every Fourth
of July, making
it a huge part
of Atlanta's
Independence
Day festivities.

exciting place to begin. The first two miles are mostly downhill. There's a temptation for newbies to go hard on this section, but we try to discourage that approach, as you'll pay for it later. On this section, you'll pass the Cathedral of St. Philip. A special moment comes when Dean Samuel G. Candler blesses passing runners by sprinkling holy water." The invocation in 2016 went as follows:

Blessings, blessings, blessings! From all over America, from all over the world, we gather this day for the blessings of running and rejoicing.

Most of us are runners, but some of us are not. Some of us are believers in God, but some of us are not. We are wheelchairs, we are walkers, we are runners, we are elite, we are not-so-elite, we are ordinary, and we are extraordinary.

But, today, we are One. We are One today, believers in the Peachtree Road Race and its ability to gather all sorts and conditions of humanity in blessing America on this Fourth of July.

Blessings to Muslims: *Assalamu alaikum!*

Blessings to Jews. *Barukh atah Adonai, Eloheinu!*

Blessings to Christians: *Christ blesses you! Benedicite Deus!*

To Hindus, to Buddhists, to atheists, to agnostics!

God blesses each and every one of us. *Dios les bendiga!*

May this Peachtree Road Race be safe and fun; may it be challenging and relaxing. May today be a holiday, a holy day, of blessing and grace, of vigor and energy!

"Once you're into mile three, you reach Cardiac Hill, which is the most famous stretch of the course," Amanda continued. "You climb twelve stories in less than a mile, and you feel it. Near the top of Cardiac Hill is the Shepherd Center, a rehabilitation clinic for patients with brain and spinal cord injuries. Some patients are out in their wheelchairs cheering participants on, which is incredibly inspiring. Some Shepherd patients also participate in our wheelchair division, which is doubly inspiring. After Cardiac Hill there are other climbs, but nothing as intense. Eventually you turn from Peachtree Road to Tenth Street. Some people think this is the end, but there's more to go. By the time you reach Tenth and Charles Allen near Piedmont Park, the race is done and you can get your race T-shirt. At most races you get your shirt when you pick up your entry materials, but not at the Peachtree. You have to finish. We hold a design contest each year for the T-shirt graphic. The public votes through the *Atlanta Journal-*

Constitution, but the winner is not revealed until race day." Refreshments and music await finishers in the park.

The success of the Peachtree owes a good deal to the ongoing support provided by Atlanta Track Club, an organization that was also cofounded by Tim Singleton. Thanks in large part to the club's leadership, Atlanta boasts one of America's largest organized running communities, with twenty-seven thousand members. The club supports high school track and field and cross-country programs around the Atlanta metropolitan area and oversees an elite team, led by Olympian Amy Begley. But the club also strives to be a resource for runners and walkers of all levels. To help less experienced runners prepare for the Peachtree, the club offers a twelve-week training program in the months leading up to the event. "We have volunteer coaches at multiple sites around the city," Amanda explained. "We call them run leads. They're present to help folks at a variety of levels, whether they are training to hit a personal record or trying to run or walk their first road race. Whatever ability level someone is at, we help them to feel confident and prepared on race day."

AMANDA KOWALESKI is the public relations and marketing communications manager at Atlanta Track Club. She has completed races ranging from 5Ks to marathons, including running the New York City Marathon for Team ASPCA to raise money for abused and neglected animals. Before coming to Atlanta Track Club, Amanda worked as a television news producer for more than a decade and for a public relations firm. She's a graduate of James Madison University.

If You Go

▶ **Getting There:** Atlanta is served by most major carriers.
▶ **Best Time to Visit:** The Peachtree Road Race is held each July 4; Atlanta Track Club holds a number of other events throughout the year.
▶ **Race Information:** Details about the Peachtree, including registration information, can be found at the Atlanta Track Club website (atlantatrackclub.org).
▶ **Accommodations:** The Atlanta Convention & Visitors Bureau (800-ATLANTA; atlanta.net) highlights a host of lodging options.

DESTINATION 22

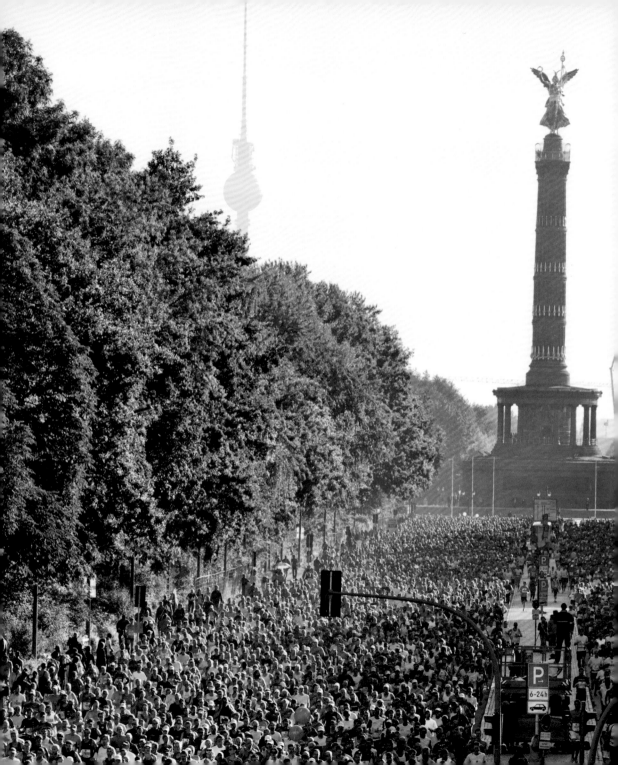

BERLIN MARATHON

RECOMMENDED BY **Thomas Steffens**

Perhaps no city in the world is more celebrated for its cultural trendsetting than Berlin. For more than a century, artists, LGBTQ individuals, and others who have struggled to fit in at home have found acceptance in the tolerant German capital. This has led to an outpouring of creativity that spans from architecture to design to a thumping late-night club scene that's likely to leave the most hardened New York club kid blushing. Berlin, it can be said, has also been on the cutting edge of road running and marathons.

"The Berlin Marathon was launched in 1974 by a group of runners from one of Germany's most prestigious athletic clubs, SC Charlottenburg," Thomas Steffens began. "The club itself dates back to the early 1900s; the first race—a cross-country race—happened in 1962. In the early years, the race was held on a minor road along the Grunewald [an area in Berlin known for its urban forest]. The first year, there were 286 starters and 244 finishers. The next few years, the race stayed small and remained on the outskirts of the city. But in September of 1981, the course was moved onto the main streets of West Berlin, beginning at the Reichstag [the former Parliament building that was famously burned in 1933] and ending on the Kurfürstendamm [a well-known avenue, considered the Champs-Elysées of Berlin.]" It was a challenge to persuade the city to allow the race to be run on public roads. The story goes that when presented with the idea by race director Horst Milde, the chief of police replied, "Roads are for cars, not for runners." But Horst prevailed, and the first men's winner was a Brit named Ian Ray, who posted a time of two hours, fifteen minutes, and forty-eight seconds; the female winner was Angelika Stephan, a German runner, with a time of two hours, forty-seven minutes, and twenty-three seconds.

"The shift to the new course through West Berlin coincided with the running boom," Thomas continued. "New York, the mother of city marathons, had popularized the idea,

OPPOSITE:
The Berlin
Marathon boasts
one of the world's
fastest marathon
courses.

111

and Stockholm was among the first in Europe to hold a large-scale race. By 1985, the race had grown to nearly ten thousand entrants." Today, the race is limited to forty thousand participants and is included in the elite World Marathon Majors series.

Many consider the BMW Berlin the world's fastest marathon track, an assertion that's reinforced by the fact that so many world records have been established on the course. (As of this writing, the most recent record was established in 2014 by Dennis Kimetto of Kenya, who completed the course in two hours, two minutes, and fifty-seven seconds.) In a story that was featured on the BBC, race director Mark Milde (son of Horst) detailed several factors that make Berlin so fast: 1) It's a flat course, with very few corners; 2) runners generally don't face a head wind; 3) the course is on asphalt, which is easier on human joints than concrete; 4) temperatures tend to be in an ideal range—between 54 and 64 degrees. In the same piece, an exercise physiologist from South Africa named Ross Tucker noted that another possible advantage is that Berlin doesn't have the budget to pay appearance fees to all the top stars. This can increase the odds of a record being broken, because when there are a number of runners vying for a record in a given race, tactical battles develop between the leaders with no one willing to sacrifice. "The optimum setup to break a world record," Ross concluded, "is to have one or two guys who are committed to going for the world record, who are willing to work together, and you just set the race up around those two."

Thomas went on to describe the course that's yielded so many world records. "One asset of the Berlin Marathon is that it starts and finishes in the same place. It's nearly in the middle of the city, and runners have great access by public transportation. The loop begins near the Brandenburg Gate, then runs past a number of Berlin landmarks—the Reichstag, the Fernsehturm [Berlin's famous TV tower, the fourth tallest structure in Europe], and Rathaus Schoneberg [once the government building that served as a backdrop for John F. Kennedy's *"Ich bin ein Berliner"* speech, now a popular flea market]. Eventually runners reach the Kurfürstendamm, passing Kaiser Wilhelm Memorial Church. At Potsdamer Platz, you cross the line where the Berlin Wall used to stand. It used to be a vast, empty area, but it was rebuilt after 1990 and is now quite fashionable. Some old sections of the wall are still visible. You'll pass Gendarmenmarkt square before coming onto Unter den Linden, a large boulevard that leads you back through the Brandenburg Gate. This stretch is very special. From the gate it's four hundred meters more to the finish line." More than a million spectators turn out each year to cheer runners on, so participants should feel plenty of encouragement.

For Thomas and many other longtime Berlin Marathon participants, the 1990 race stands out as a watershed moment. "The marathon always happens in September," he recalled, "and that year, the Berlin Wall had come down just a few months earlier. East Germany still existed [reunification would occur a few days later, on October 3], though there were no real controls at the border. When the wall came down, the race organizers decided that the course would have to be altered to include East Berlin. The start was moved to a point a few kilometers before the Brandenburg Gate. It would head about 3.5 kilometers through Tiergarten park and then pass through the gate. Before the route change was announced, the race had seventeen thousand entrants. When people realized it was going through the Brandenburg Gate, participation immediately swelled to twenty-five thousand, which was the upper limit; we could have filled fifty thousand spots. I didn't run the entire race that year, as I was injured, but I did run the first ten miles. Passing through the gate was incredibly emotional."

The female winner that year, incidentally, was Uta Pippig—from East Germany.

THOMAS STEFFENS is a former journalist, the founding editor of *Runner's World*, German edition, and an author of several running books. Since 2007 he has been the spokesperson for the Berlin Marathon. He has run twenty-five marathons in Europe and the United States.

23

DESTINATION

If You Go

▶ **Getting There:** Berlin is served by most major international carriers.

▶ **Best Time to Visit:** The BMW Berlin Marathon is generally run the fourth Sunday in September.

▶ **Race Information:** Everything you need to know about the Berlin Marathon (including registration information) resides at bmw-berlin-marathon.com/en.

▶ **Accommodations:** Visit Berlin (+49 03025002333; visitberlin.de) lists lodging options throughout the city.

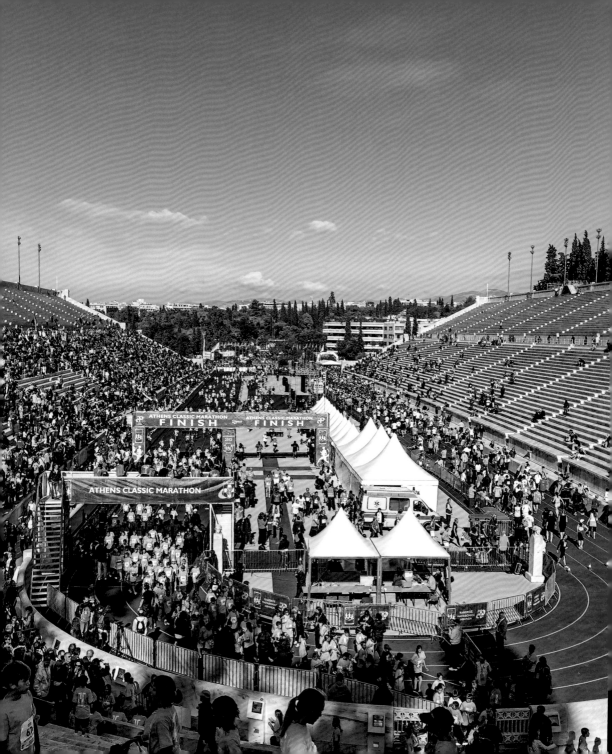

ATHENS MARATHON

RECOMMENDED BY **Paul Samaras**

When the first "marathon" was run, there was no prize money on the line, no sponsor products to peddle, no personal bests or world records hanging in the balance. Instead, it was the very idea of democracy. "At the time, 490 BCE, *dēmokratía* was still a revolutionary and novel concept," Paul Samaras began. "The idea of 'rule of the people' had been born less than a generation before, and the Battle of Marathon—which pitted the Athenians against the Persians—was its first true test, fought by free Athenian men. As legend has it, a courier named Pheidippides—the fastest man among the Athenian soldiers—ran from the battlefields at Marathon to alert the citizens of Athens that their army had prevailed, and died after sharing his news. It became symbolic of the victory of democracy and much later served as the model for the long-distance run in the first modern Olympics. Many runners long to make the pilgrimage to compete in the Athens Marathon, as golfers want to visit St. Andrews in Scotland. This is where it began, and they want to run the original course. I've had a number of first-time marathon runners visit over the years. Their thinking is, 'If I'm going to run a marathon, I may as well start with the first.'"

The first modern Olympic Games were staged in 1896 in Athens. The revival can be largely credited to a Frenchman named Pierre de Coubertin, who idealized ancient Greece and advocated for the benefits of physical education. He saw the revitalization of an international Olympic Games as a means to promote better understanding among cultures, and as an opportunity to stress the importance of struggle and competition, rather than winning. Another Frenchman (and comrade of Pierre), Michel Bréal, is frequently cited as the inventor of the modern marathon; he is said to have based the course for the first Olympic marathon on the purported route of Pheidippides. (The exact route that Pheidippides took—and even whether the courier was named Pheidippides—is

OPPOSITE:
The Athens
Marathon
closely follows
the course that
historians believe
Pheidippides took
in 490 BCE.
It ends in the
Olympic stadium,
which was erected
in 1896.

24

DESTINATION

somewhat in question. Another story goes that the courier—named Philippides in some accounts—ran from Marathon to Sparta, a distance of nearly 150 miles, more than two days' time, in an attempt to rally forces . . . but the Spartans were unable to leave until a religious festival had finished, and hence he ran back.) The winner of the first Olympic marathon was Greek runner Spyridon Louis, who emerged victorious from a field of seventeen, nine of whom finished. His winning time was two hours, fifty-eight minutes, and fifty seconds. The course at that time was forty kilometers, or just under twenty-five miles. The last 1.2 miles weren't added to the standard marathon distance until the London Olympics in 1908; originally from Windsor Castle to White City Stadium, the London course traversed twenty-six miles—plus an extra 385 yards inside the stadium to take participants past the royal viewing box.

It should be noted that in the ancient Olympics, which date back to 776 BCE, there was no marathon. The longest running event, the *dolichos*, maxed out at 4,800 meters.

The current Athens Marathon course has been extended to 26.2 miles and moves in a generally westward direction from the town of Marathon. "It's the same course that was used in the 2004 Olympics," Paul continued, "and according to historians that were involved, it closely follows the path that a runner would have taken from Marathon to Athens. It's hard not to feel that you're running in the footsteps of heroes from classical times. One of the special moments comes after three or four kilometers, when runners take a detour off the course and circle the earth mound tomb of the fallen Athenians. This rests at the site of an actual battleground and commemorates the sacrifice of 192 Athenian soldiers. From here, the course goes southwest and then bends northwest, passing through farmland and small towns. Many of the local people come out on the day of the marathon, clapping and encouraging the runners along. Some will hand olive branches to runners as motivation. The tradition of the olive branch goes back to the first Olympics of 776 BCE. There was a sacred olive tree next to the Temple of Zeus (one of the seven wonders of the ancient world). Branches were cut from the tree and fashioned into wreaths for the winners of each event. Victors would also receive a ceramic pot bearing an illustration of the event that they'd won; the pot was filled with olive oil made from the olives of the sacred tree. Many associate the Olympics with laurel wreaths, but the tradition of using laurel branches came later, at the games held in Delphi."

As runners reach the outskirts of Athens, they'll pass another landmark, the two-story sculpture of the runner. "It's very modernist, with thick panes of glass stacked atop each other to create the likeness of a windswept runner," Paul described. "As you get closer to the city, you'll catch a glimpse of the Acropolis, which is the hill on which the Parthenon rests. Part of the Parthenon is blocked out by the stadium, but it's visible. This is very moving for runners, as it's one of the most recognizable buildings in the world, and stands for democracy and individual spirit. It was built to last as a reminder of what a handful of people were able to create." The race ends in the Olympic stadium first built to house the 1896 games.

"When everyone has finished, we take our runners back to our hotel for a formal dinner," Paul added. "After a four-course meal, we have presentations and Greek dancers, and each runner is presented with an olive wreath that my family members who live in Greece have made. Runners also receive a miniature ceramic vase, similar to what they would have received had they competed in the first Olympic Games."

PAUL SAMARAS has specialized in support packages for the Athens Marathon since 1994. Since 1995, he has worked closely with the organizing committee, SEGAS (Hellenic Amateur Athletic Association), on the race. A retired businessman and former restaurateur, Paul now lives in Denver and is the owner of Apostolos Greek Tours (athensmarathon.com).

If You Go

▶ **Getting There:** Athens is served by most major international carriers.
▶ **Best Time to Visit:** The Athens Marathon is generally held on the second Sunday of November each year.
▶ **Race Information:** The Athens Marathon organizing committee website (athens authenticmarathon.gr) details the event. Apostolos Greek Tours (303-755-2888; athensmarathon.com) offers several marathon tour packages that include race registration and support, lodging, and sight-seeing.
▶ **Accommodations:** The Greek National Tourism Organization (visitgreece.gr) lists lodging options around Athens.

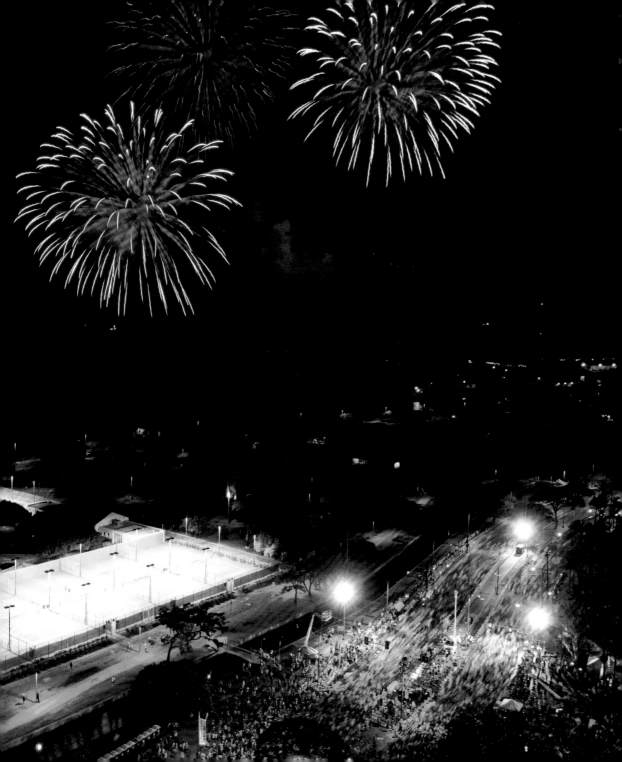

HONOLULU MARATHON

RECOMMENDED BY **Jim Barahal**

Marathons are, on one level, about competition. Elite runners compete with one another for prize money and bragging rights. The vast majority of marathoners compete with themselves. The Honolulu Marathon attracts many elites to the island of Oahu each December, but for Jim Barahal, it's always been about individual accomplishment. "I see the Honolulu Marathon as a great venue for participatory fun. The course has many scenic vistas. It's challenging, but not ridiculous. You can make it whatever you want it to be, as competitive as you want to make it. Everyone is an athlete, whatever your time. I feel that in putting the race on, it's our role to provide a canvas for individual runners to paint their own picture. We let people define their own accomplishment."

The Honolulu Marathon is among America's oldest marathons, first run in 1973. That year, there were 162 entrants and 151 finishers. By 2016, the event had ballooned to more than thirty-three thousand runners, with nearly half traveling to Oahu from Japan. (In Japan, there are relatively few marathons open to all comers, hence the appeal of this race.) The event was championed by then Honolulu mayor Frank Fasi, who wrote, "Having been born and raised in New England, I have long been impressed by the magnitude and success of the famous run in Boston. It seems to me that Honolulu could well host such an event, considering local interest and our location in the Pacific area." Mayor Fasi's enthusiasm for the event was reinforced by a local cardiologist named Jack Scaff, who early on recognized the potential of running as therapy for heart disease . . . a revelation that helped accelerate the running craze of the seventies.

From its inception, the Honolulu Marathon has had no cutoff time for runners. "Many big marathons are built to maximize performance," Jim continued. "They're run in the spring or fall, so temperatures are between 48 and 58 degrees. In Hawaii, you're

OPPOSITE:
Fireworks
celebrate the
five A.M. *start*
of the Honolulu
Marathon.

not ever going to get optimal conditions; it's too warm. That changes the nature of the activity. It becomes more of party, a festival environment." When the Honolulu Marathon organizers state that there's not a cutoff time, they mean it—in 2013, the last participant crossed the finish line in Kapiolani Park nineteen hours, thirty-nine minutes, and thirty-four seconds after the start.

While the course and conditions in Honolulu may not be conducive to personal bests, most marathoners will agree that the race is among the most scenic you'll find anywhere. Jim summarized the route. "The race begins at five A.M., in Ala Moana Beach Park—the early start is a nod to giving runners a bit of a performance edge. It's very theatrical, as we have ten minutes of fireworks. You almost feel like you're on a movie set. From the park, runners loop through the downtown area, past Iolani Palace and city hall. Many of the buildings have Christmas lights up, which adds to the festive atmosphere. Around the six-mile mark, you come into Waikiki. Though it's still early, there are a lot of people out cheering you on. Soon after, you come to Diamond Head [a volcanic cone that is 762 feet at its highest point], which involves a pretty significant climb. For a lot of runners, there's a level of euphoric energy that comes with a mass marathon—irrational exuberance, if you will. At the Diamond Head climb, some of this exuberance diminishes. You still have eighteen miles to go, and you realize that this might be a little harder than you thought.

"After passing Diamond Head, you head inland for a few miles before returning to the coast by Waialae Country Club. The next four miles you're on Kalanianaole Highway. As the sky lightens (for runners of average pace), you'll see Koko Head Crater in the distance. (For the elite runners, the sun is rising as they climb Diamond Head the second time at mile twenty-four.) At Maunalua Bay you head inland a bit and turn to loop back. The last eight miles are all along the water. It's another tough climb as you pass Diamond Head again, but you can suck it up because you're almost done, and there's a downhill on the other side. The finish is at Kapiolani Park." Treats at the Finisher's Food Court include *malasadas*, a kind of hole-less doughnut that was originally brought to Hawaii by Portuguese laborers in the late nineteenth century.

Given Honolulu's emphasis on individual accomplishment—no matter how that's defined—Jim has at times wondered whether professional runners belong in the race. The answer has always been "Yes!" "I think it's a big deal to see the leaders, to see people who are tops in the world in action," Jim opined. "At most big races, there's a good chance that folks who are toward the middle or the back of the pack won't set eyes on the leading racers at all. The way Honolulu is set up, the elite runners are coming back toward the finish while many racers are making their way to the turn. People who are toward the back may be at mile seven, and they'll be within five feet of the winner as he heads into mile twenty-six. I think this connects average runners to top runners.

"Running a marathon has a clock on it, which gives it objectivity and fosters comparison. However, I think most runners are doing it for themselves. It's for you. We all go through different phases in our running, and I think it's important to give ourselves the flexibility to redefine our accomplishments as we move along. I stand at the finish line at the eight-hour mark and watch people coming in and see their joy. This reminds me of why they're doing it. And why I'm still involved."

JIM BARAHAL has been the president of the Honolulu Marathon since 1988. Since taking over the event in 1987, he has developed the race into one of the world's largest marathons and the sporting event with the biggest economic impact in Hawaii. Jim grew up in Detroit; after coming to Hawaii in 1979, he quickly became one the islands' top runners, as he had trained with the University of Michigan track team while in med school. In addition to his work on the Honolulu Marathon, Jim has directed financial support of youth sporting events like the Honolulu Marathon/HHSAA Cross Country Championships and the Honolulu Marathon Track and Field Invitational. In 2015, he was inducted into the Hawaii Sports Hall of Fame.

If You Go

► **Getting There:** Oahu (Honolulu) is served by most major carriers.
► **Best Time to Visit:** The Honolulu Marathon is generally held on the second Sunday in December.
► **Race Information:** Details, including registration information, are available at honolulu marathon.org.
► **Accommodations:** Outrigger Hotels & Resorts (866-956-4262; outrigger.com) is the official hotel group of the Honolulu Marathon. The Oahu Visitors Bureau (visit-oahu. com) provides an overview of the many lodging options around Honolulu.

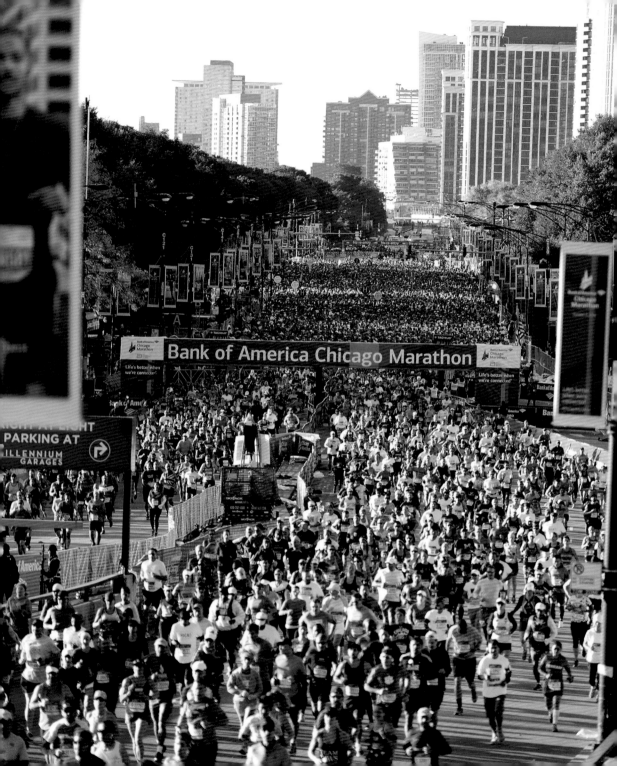

CHICAGO MARATHON

RECOMMENDED BY **Peter Sagal**

When Peter Sagal saw a shadowy figure clad in a black cloak and bearing a scythe in the distance, he did what any sane person would do—he started to run.

"I had run cross-country in high school in New Jersey," Peter began. "But as I got older, I slowed down a bit. As I was turning forty, I had a classic midlife crisis. I thought, 'Now I'm going to die . . . but if I run a marathon, I won't die.' I tried to train up in 2005 to see if I could finish the Chicago Marathon, as I live in Chicago now. I found a plan online and tried to keep with it. Unfortunately, I didn't start slowly enough and injured myself, which led to me missing more than a month of training in the middle. I wondered if I should go through with it, but as I'd told everyone that I was going to run, I had to. I made many of the mistakes one could make in running their first marathon, but I finished in four hours and three minutes. I thought that I'd be done with it. But as time passed, I became interested in seeing if I could improve on my first time. Since then, I've become a serious runner . . . and I eventually cut almost an hour off my original time."

The Chicago Marathon as we know it today was first conceived of in November of 1976, by five Chicagolanders: Wayne Goeldner, physical education director of the Hyde Park YMCA; Wendell "Wendy" Miller, a partner in a financial advising firm and founder of Midwest Masters Running Club; Bill Robinson, executive director of Friends of the Parks; Sharon Mier, director of women's sports at the Loop Center YMCA; and Dr. Noel Nequin, director of cardiac rehabilitation at Swedish Covenant Hospital. Although plans for the marathon were slow to materialize, Dr. Nequin was able to organize a ten-mile run, the Ravenswood Bank Lakefront, in May of 1977. The race had been expected to attract three hundred runners, but one thousand showed up—including then Chicago mayor Michael Bilandic, who liked to run. His interest in a longer run was piqued—and as often is the case

OPPOSITE:
The Chicago
Marathon
celebrated
its fortieth
anniversary
in 2017 and
now attracts
forty-five
thousand
runners.

DESTINATION

26

in the Windy City, a little interest from the mayor goes a long way. Chicago's inaugural marathon was held on September 25, 1977, attracting more than 4,200 participants, thus making it the world's largest marathon to that date.

These days, the Bank of America Chicago Marathon limits participation to forty-five thousand runners and is classified as one of the six World Marathon Majors.

"I've run a number of different urban marathons," Peter continued. "Chicago offers a tremendous course. For starters, it's very convenient, starting and ending right at the lakefront [at Grant Park]. You don't have to get yourself to a faraway starting point. The way the course is set up offers a wonderful tour of the city's neighborhoods. [The course visits twenty-nine neighborhoods in all.] And it takes you past many Chicago landmarks—among them the Loop, Wrigley Field, and Chinatown. Plus, it's flat as a pancake." (This last facet of the race has made Chicago the site of more than a few world and national records over the years . . . not to mention a multitude of personal bests.)

"The first half of the race is fantastic," Peter continued. "You're running north through the Loop, and the crowds are out. You head through the canyon of LaSalle Street and then up toward Lincoln Park. By the time you reach Boystown, the streets are packed. [Attendance in 2016 was estimated at 1.7 million.] There are cheerleaders and rock bands playing. You continue out to the West Side, where you'll pass the United Center [home of the Chicago Bulls and Blackhawks]. From here you begin to head back downtown. You'll run through some of the older ethnic neighborhoods—Little Italy, Greektown, then Chinatown, where there are dragon dancers to cheer you on. Not long after comes the toughest stretch. Many marathon courses begin by taking runners past less interesting areas and conclude with the most exciting spots. Chicago does the opposite. With six miles to go, you reach the most desolate part of the course. It's a post-industrial stretch along Interstate 94, 1.5 miles that test runners' souls. I actually wrote a short play about that stretch. But like any good drama, things soon improve. First comes Bronzeville, then the Illinois Institute of Technology campus. When you turn onto Michigan Avenue, you can hear the crowds. From here, it's a final dash to a right turn on Roosevelt Road, and then a left turn to the finish back at Grant Park. I'll never forget the 2006 race. I was hoping to qualify for the Boston Marathon, and I was on pace to do so. Then I got a cramp on Michigan Avenue. I was terrified, but I made it by nineteen seconds!"

No reflection on the Chicago running scene would be complete without mention of the Lakefront Trail, an eighteen-mile stretch along Lake Michigan that has encouraged tens of thousands of Chicagoans to get out and run.

PETER SAGAL left Berkeley Heights, New Jersey, to attend Harvard University and subsequently squandered that education while working as a literary manager for a regional theater, a movie publicist, a stage director, an actor, an extra in a Michael Jackson video, a travel writer, an essayist, a ghostwriter for a former adult film impresario, and a staff writer for a motorcycle magazine. He is the author of numerous plays that have been performed in large and small theaters around the country and abroad. Peter has also written a number of screenplays, including *Savage*, a cheesy vehicle for obscure French kickboxer Olivier Gruner, and *Cuba Mine*, an original screenplay that became, without his knowledge, the basis for *Dirty Dancing: Havana Nights*. Among Peter's honors in the theater are a Drama-Logue Award for directing, grants from the Jerome and McKnight Foundations, and a residency grant at the Camargo Foundation in Cassis, France. In 1997, Peter joined the panel of a news quiz show on NPR, coproduced by WBEZ Chicago, which made its debut on-air in January of 1998. In May of that year, he moved to Chicago to become the host of the show. Since then, *Wait Wait . . . Don't Tell Me!* has become one of the most popular shows on public radio, heard by nearly three million listeners on 520 public radio stations nationwide and by a million people every month via podcast. He is also the author of *The Book of Vice: Very Naughty Things (and How to Do Them)* and a book about running to be published by Simon and Schuster.

If You Go

▶ **Getting There:** Chicago is served by most major carriers.
▶ **Best Time to Visit:** The Bank of America Chicago Marathon is held in early October.
▶ **Race Information:** The Chicago Marathon website (chicagomarathon.com) covers all the details you need to participate (including how to apply). Though spots fill up fast, some slots are available for latecomers through charity organizations.
▶ **Accommodations:** The Chicago Hilton (855-760-0869; hilton.com) is the official hotel of the marathon. Other options are highlighted at Choose Chicago (choosechicago.com).

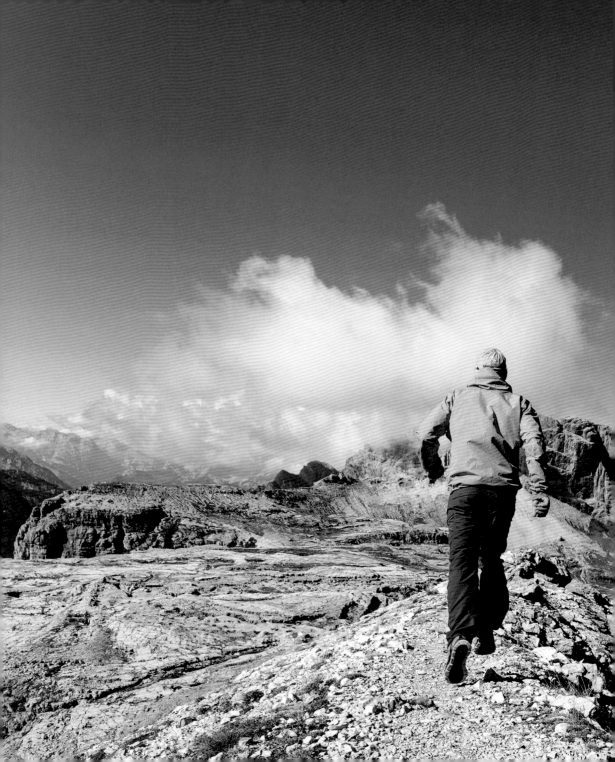

THE DOLOMITES

RECOMMENDED BY **Jeremy Wolf**

"The Dolomites stand out to me as a stunning mountain range, with jagged peaks that stretch into an incredibly blue sky and drop into compact, verdant valleys," Jeremy Wolf began. "When you're at the top of a portion of trail, you're not looking fifty miles across. Your views are condensed to the valley below. From a trail-running perspective, the terrain is very appealing—you run up one mountain, then down into a steep valley. There's great diversity of terrain in a compact area. Another great aspect of the Dolomites is the system of trails and rifugios. [Rifugios are lodgings that range from boutique inns to bed-and-breakfasts to hostels.] The massive trail network was built largely during World War I to assist the Italians in their battle against the Austrian-Hungarians. As you're running, you see many remnants of the war effort—tunnels, bunkers, stone forts; it's a history tour as well as a trail run. The rifugio network is one of the keys to making long-distance trail running in the Dolomites work. The rifugios were designed to support day hikers, so they're spaced with regularity along the trail system. They provide fine meals, plus comfortable beds for the night. As a trail runner, the presence of the rifugios means you can travel extremely light. There's no need to carry food, sleeping bags, tents, etc."

Jeremy and his two longtime running mates—Jason Schlarb and Matt Lowe—began their run in the village of Calalzo, roughly one hundred miles north of Venice. Their plan was to cover some ninety miles over five days, ending their journey in Cortina. "We planned the trip on our own," Jeremy continued, "and the resources from Club Alpino Italiano, plus the knowledge shared by the rifugio owners, made it possible. We began our run on June 10. On an average year, most of the trails would be clear of snow, but it had been very cold in Europe that winter, and the Dolomites had a record level of snow in places. We weren't expecting the amount of snow we experienced on the route. This

OPPOSITE:
The Dolomites'
incredible beauty
and intricate
system of
rifugios make
them ideal for
trail running
odysseys.

DESTINATION

27

added a level of excitement and nervousness to the run, as we didn't know from one day to the next whether we'd be able to follow the route we'd mapped out. We were relying on our rifugio hosts to tell us what routes to take; they were kind enough to call ahead to the next rifugio on the trail and check how conditions were. There were a few times when we were told that a trail was not passable. Rightfully or wrongfully, we attempted the trail anyway. Every time, we were able to navigate it." One positive of the snow was that Jeremy, Jason, and Matt had little trouble finding space when they reached their rifugio of choice. "When we'd come into some of the rifugios, they'd ask where we came from," Jeremy added. "When we told them, the response would be, 'Ah! You opened the route!' "

The route that the trio chose started in a generally northerly direction before heading west and then south to Cortina. "There are a hundred different routes a runner could take, and they all have something to offer," Jeremy described. "There are enough little roads in the Dolomites that you can find a way out when you're done running." The group covered between twenty-one and thirty miles a day, including up to eight thousand feet of elevation gain . . . much of this scrambling over snow. "It was a pretty simple schedule," Jeremy continued. "We'd wake up in the morning and have a hearty breakfast. It might be cured meats, cheeses, and grapes. You could ask for a lunch to be prepared, and then you'd be off. We carried long-sleeve shirts and pants, sunglasses, and some snacks. Some days we'd stop for lunch at a rifugio along the way. The trails—when we could locate them—took us on ridgelines, down steep declines into mountain meadows, and then up again. The scenery was tremendous throughout the run. One highlight was certainly Tre Cime, three giant rock towers with flat vertical faces that jut out from the surrounding peaks. Another was reaching Strudelkopf Peak, which has 360-degree views of the Dolomites . . . including Tre Cime across the valley. When we'd get to the rifugio where we planned to stay, we'd get a shower and then dinner. The rifugios were near the tops of the passes and had tremendous views. On our second night, at a rifugio called Auronzo, Tre Cime was right before us. As for the food, it was very local—some more Italian, some more Germanic depending on where we were. Each region has its own grappa, an Italian brandy made from wine, and there was also Italian beer. Our hosts didn't always speak English, but all were very friendly. I thought the food was very good, though it didn't really matter. We were trying to get every calorie we could."

The Alta Vias (public footpaths) that were built in the Dolomites during World War I traverse some precipitous terrain. While the alpine ibex (wild goats) that flourish here need little assistance, humans will find assistance from via ferratas that dot the trails. A via ferrata ("iron road" in Italian) is a series of rungs, rails, and/or cables that permit travelers to scale rock faces that might otherwise be too steep. One of Jeremy's most memorable moments of his run through the Dolomites came on his last day, when he and his mates discovered Via Ferrata Lucio Dalaiti. "We saw the steel rungs in the side of the cliff and thought, 'This looks amazing,'" he recalled. "We took it down to the amazing eighty-foot waterfall. The trail actually went behind it. You could feel its thundering inside your bones. We continued down to another even taller waterfall. That mile or two was full of adventure and excitement. It captured the essence of mountain climbing and trail running."

JEREMY WOLF ran collegiate track and cross-country at Montana State University. He is a founding member of Montana Trail Crew, a trail-running advocacy organization, and he directs the Mountain Running Film Festival. With Schlarb-Wolf Productions (schlarb wolf.com), Jeremy produces films of his international running adventures, including *Opening the Route*, set in the Italian Dolomites, and *Around Patagonia*. His sponsors include HOKA ONE ONE, Ultimate Direction, and Julbo Eyewear. Jeremy takes in views of the Rocky Mountains from his office as a business and engineering consultant in Missoula, Montana.

If You Go

▶ **Getting There:** The route that Jeremy chose is most easily reached from Venice, which is served by most major carriers.
▶ **Best Time to Visit:** The Dolomites are best run between June 15 and October 15 . . . though some years, the snow can linger into later June.
▶ **Running Information:** Club Alpino Italiano (cai.it) is a starting point for maps and suggested routes.
▶ **Accommodations:** There are many rifugios spread throughout the Dolomites, usually within five to ten miles of each other. Most have websites. Rifugio Auronzo (rifugio auronzo.it), Rifugio Vallandro (vallandro.it/eng), and Rifugio Lavarella (lavarella.it) are a few that Jeremy visited.

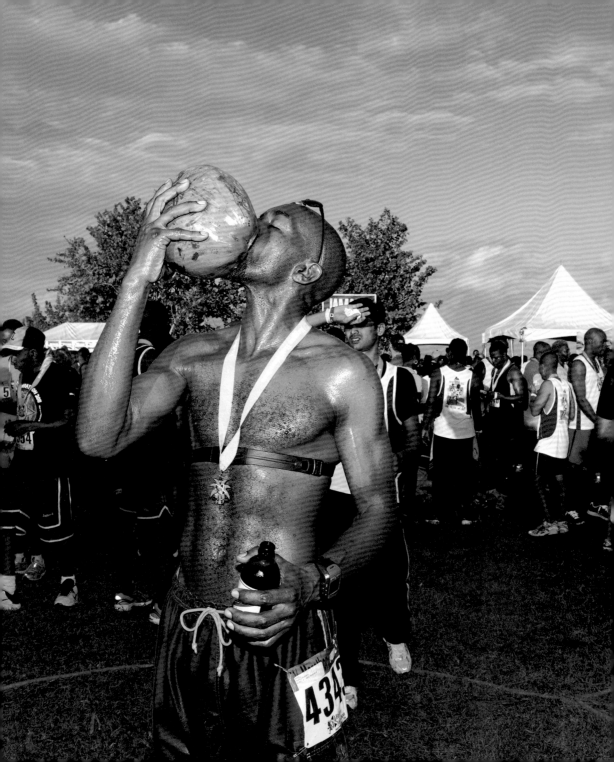

REGGAE MARATHON

RECOMMENDED BY **Alfred Francis**

At the beginning of "Trenchtown Rock" (1975), Bob Marley sings:

One good thing about music, when it hits you feel no pain
One good thing about music, when it hits you feel no pain
So hit me with music, hit me with music
Hit me with music, hit me with music now

If you believe that music—especially good reggae music—can help ease the soreness and fatigue of a long-distance run, you might consider a trip to Negril, Jamaica, to participate in the Reggae Marathon.

"There is a group of long-distance runners based in Kingston called the Jamdammers," Alfred Francis began. (The name stems from their original gathering spot, a reservoir called Mona Dam, known locally as the Dam.) "We had all run marathons in other places before. A few of us went to the Rock 'n' Roll Marathon in San Diego and had the idea we should put on a big marathon in Jamaica, taking advantage of our music, food, and that special Jamaican vibe. We knew the perfect spot: Negril, a beach community on the west side of the island. Early December is a shoulder season there, so bringing in visitors would help the local economy. We approached Rita Marley [the late Bob Marley's wife] and asked if we could use her and Bob's names on the trophies. She kindly consented, and we commissioned a noted Jamaican sculptor, Basil Watson, to create the Bob Marley Trophy for the male winner and the Rita Marley Trophy for the female winner." The first Reggae Marathon (which also includes a half marathon and 10K) was held in 2001.

OPPOSITE:
A runner enjoys some fresh coconut water (and a Red Stripe beer) at the Reggae Marathon.

DESTINATION

28

131

(The notion that reggae music might help a runner's pacing has some scientific validity. A study published in the British Medical Journal publication *Heart* showed that listening to slower music resulted in a significant drop in heart rate and blood pressure. Reggae music brought about the largest decline in heart rate of the musical styles used in the study.)

Negril, the setting for the Reggae Marathon, fits central casting's criteria for "idyllic Caribbean hideaway." The village's main attraction is its seven-mile beach of powdery white sand, dotted with requisite coconut palms, sloping gently down to the placid hot-tub-warm sea. In the sixties, "flower children" were drawn to the beach, the music, and the availability of ganja in Negril. Since that time, it has slowly evolved to embrace more conventional beach tourism while still managing to evade the kind of overdevelopment that would jeopardize its signature ambiance.

The festivities surrounding the Reggae Marathon begin with the Friday night pasta feed—in some estimations, the world's best pre-run pasta event. "We have all the wonderful hotels in the village come with a variety of their best pasta dishes," Alfred continued. "It's truly a culinary delight. Some years we'll have the dinner on the beach, as the sun sets. Of course, there's music too." As tempting as it might be to let the revelry stretch far into the evening, runners will do well to turn in early, as the Reggae Marathon has one of the running world's earliest starts—5:15 A.M. "It's a truly wonderful start at Long Bay Beach Park," Alfred described. "Torchbearers raise bamboo torches, and Bob Marley songs play—'Jammin' ' or 'One Love.' The temperature is a comfortable 76 degrees (one reason for the early start), and runners do the first few miles in the moonlight. The mostly flat course follows the beach out, with Long Bay to the west, then loops into the town of Negril before heading toward the town of Green Island and returning to the park. The marathon runners do two loops; the half marathoners run one; and the 10K runners do half a loop. Music is a mainstay of the run, and we have some sort of music every eight hundred meters along the course—full live bands, drummers, or steel drummers, as well as sound systems playing Bob Marley so you can run to the rhythm.

"When runners reach the finish at the park, there's coconut water waiting, loads of Red Stripe beer, and a host of fresh fruit. Most runners will head right to the beach, just four hundred meters away. Here, there are two huge tents where you can get a massage. Many will wade right into the warm sea, which has therapeutic qualities. Of course, the music continues. For entertainment we feature up-and-coming reggae acts."

Though it's modest in size relative to many marathons—participation maxes out at three thousand and is typically a bit lower—the Reggae Marathon gets consistently high marks for its excellent execution. This is in large part thanks to the Jamdammers who volunteer to man the race. "All the Jamdammers have run marathons and understand what the runners are going through," Francis explained. Even though we have a course limit for marathoners (six hours), we disregard it if a person is within two miles. We won't close the course in those cases, even if we have to wait eight hours. We've even brought music out to help bring them home."

Jamaica has made a name in the track and field industry by producing the world's fastest sprinters—most recently Usain Bolt and Elaine Thompson. Will a time come when the world's greatest distance runners also hail from this Caribbean island? "I don't think we have any Usain Bolts in the marathon category in the near-term," Francis opined. "But we are working on laying the foundation for them to emerge."

ALFRED "FRANO" FRANCIS is the race director of the Reggae Marathon. He and his Running Events Limited team, along with the Jamdammers, operate twenty races annually in Jamaica, including the Sagicor Sigma Corporate Run, the Tru-Juice Run For Your Cause, the CUMI Come Run, Digicel's Night Run, and the CB Group/UWI 5K Run/Walk. In 2014, Alfred was awarded the national honor of the Order of Distinction in recognition of his contribution to the fitness and healthy-lifestyle landscape in Jamaica.

DESTINATION

28

If You Go

▶ **Getting There:** Most visitors to Negril fly into Montego Bay, which is served by a number of carriers, including Delta (800-221-1212; delta.com) and United (800-864-8331; united.com).

▶ **Best Time to Visit:** The Reggae Marathon is held in early December.

▶ **Race Information:** All you need to know about the Reggae Marathon, including registration details, resides at reggaemarathon.com.

▶ **Accommodations:** The Reggae Marathon website lists a number of options around Negril; more options can be found at the Jamaica Tourist Board site (visitjamaica.com) and the Negril Chamber of Commerce site (negrilchamberofcommerce.com).

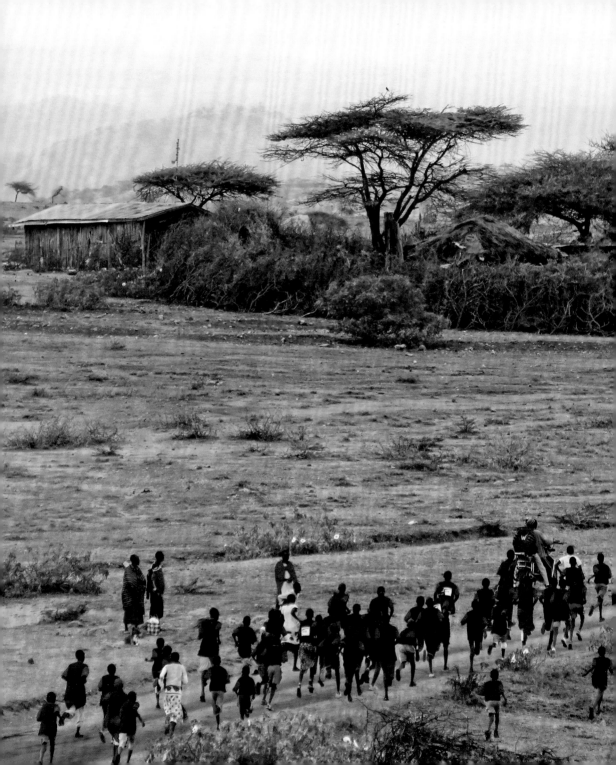

AMAZING MAASAI MARATHON

RECOMMENDED BY **Jacqui Kaufman**

"I've led tours to marathons around the world," Jacqui Kaufman began, "and on those tours, people often ask me if there's only one trip I could do, which would it be? I never hesitate—it's the Amazing Maasai Marathon in Kenya. I also advise people that it could very well be life changing. It certainly was for me."

The Maasai Mara National Reserve rests in the southwest corner of Kenya, just north of the Serengeti National Park in Tanzania; it's the northern edge of the greater Mara-Serengeti ecosystem. It's home to a rich assemblage of the animal life that people travel to Africa to experience on safari—including lions, leopards, cheetahs, Cape buffalo, elephants, rhinoceroses, hippopotamuses, and crocodiles. The location also figures in one of the animal world's great point-to-point marathons—the Great Migration—when zebras, wildebeests, and Thomson's gazelles move from the Serengeti to the Maasai Mara (in July) and back (in October). The region is also known for its eponymous Maasai people, whose nomadic, pastoral culture has traditionally relied on cattle herds for sustenance.

"If I were to write a book about Kenya, it would be titled *Africa: It's Not What You Think*," Jacqui continued. "For example, when I tell people in Colorado that I'm going to run a marathon in Kenya in July or August, their first response is, 'Goodness, it will be so hot!' The reality is, it's cooler than Boulder is at that time. People also have the perception that Kenya is not safe. That may be true of parts of Nairobi, but it's certainly not the case in the countryside. I've always found that the Kenyan people were warm and friendly. And the animals—that may be the main reason to do this trip. On the animal viewing portions of the trip, you feel like you've wandered onto a *National Geographic* set. You're riding in a jeep with no boundaries and no fences. At times, there are animals as far as you can see. Elephants, lions, the herd animals, maybe leopards and cheetahs. There's

OPPOSITE:
During the Amazing Maasai Marathon, many local children will join in for sections of the race.

DESTINATION

29

135

such a sense of privilege to be with these animals on their land." Jacqui was particularly taken with the African lions and their amazing social behavior. On returning home, she felt compelled to learn more about lions and subsequently became involved with a rehabilitation program in Zimbabwe for young lions.

The Amazing Maasai Marathon came into being thanks to a television show filmed far away in China. There, while making *The Amazing Race: China Rush*, two American ultramarathoners met two Maasai runners. Though the four were technically competing against each other, they became fast friends. Their conversations led to the idea of starting an endurance race in Kenya to raise money so that Maasai girls could go to school. This led to the creation of the Amazing Maasai Girls Project, which manages the race. All donations and proceeds from the marathon (and accompanying half marathon) go toward the sponsorship of Maasai girls through secondary school. As of this writing, more than $180,000 has been raised, and more than sixty girls have received (or are receiving) an education.

The race is held in and around the village of Kimanjo, which rests in the lower Rift Valley. The dirt track loop course winds through long (though not terrifically steep) hills, flat bushlands, and rolling countryside. It's at altitude—roughly five thousand feet—but visitors will have had a few days to acclimatize to the elevation. "You don't see any of the region's wild animals on the course, though you do see camels occasionally," Jacqui observed. (To prevent any unwelcome encounters, the course is patrolled by experienced, military-trained scouts who track the animals and their movements.) "For parts of the run, young Maasai kids will run with you. It's the event of the year for the community, this race when the *mozunga* (white people) come. One year, I must have run thirty minutes with two kids on either side of me, holding my hands. They'll do this with all the runners. On another occasion, I saw a Maasai warrior standing on a hillside as I ran by—it was almost surreal. It's always very special to be running through an ancient culture, so far removed from our life in America."

Like most Marathon Tours expeditions, the Amazing Maasai adventure is as much about the path to the run as the run itself. "After a night in Nairobi, we head to Aberdare National Park," Jacqui described. "Here we have our first game drive. There's a watering hole at the lodge where we stay with a wooden structure built nearby. You can observe elephants, buffalo, sometimes hyenas. The next day there's the option to take a practice run with a local guide, to help you acclimatize to the elevation (roughly seven thousand feet at Aberdare Hills). You're running among giraffes, zebras, and other wildlife within the conservancy. Then we move on to Sweetwaters Tented Camp in the Ol Pejeta Conservancy for several days. Here, there are several days with more opportunities for game drives, and another watering hole at the camp where you can watch game as the sun sets. You'll then move on to Kimanjo, where you'll have a chance to visit one of the schools that the marathon benefits.

"I just can't say enough about the experience. The air, the smell of the grasslands, the Maasai girls in their traditional garb, the animals roaming free, the sunrises and sunsets. It's always such a privilege."

JACQUI KAUFMAN was born and raised in Great Britain and has worked on and off in the travel industry for more than twenty years. She has traveled extensively and lived in numerous countries around the world including United Arab Emirates, South Africa, Indonesia, and Uruguay before settling in the United States in 1980. Passionate about running and adventure, Jacqui has completed more than fifty marathons and has competed in ultra events such as the Leadville 100, the Himalayan Stage Race, Alaska's Iditasport 100 and 350, and the Yukon Arctic Ultra, to name a few. Addicted to the outdoors, Jacqui lives in Boulder, Colorado, where she enjoys trail running, hiking, climbing, winter sports, and yoga. She will always remember spending several summers rehabilitating lions in Zimbabwe with ALERT.

DESTINATION

29

If You Go

▶ **Getting There:** Most international travelers will fly into Nairobi, which is served by many major carriers. Those traveling with a tour will take a charter flight from the Maasai Mara to Kimanjo and then back to Nairobi.

▶ **Best Time to Visit:** The Amazing Maasai Marathon is generally held in late July, when temperatures are fairly mild.

▶ **Race Information:** An overview of the Amazing Maasai Marathon resides at amazingmaasaimarathon.com. Most participants will choose to run this event with a tour company like Marathon Tours & Travel (617-242-7845; marathontours.com), which takes care of registration, transportation, and accommodations.

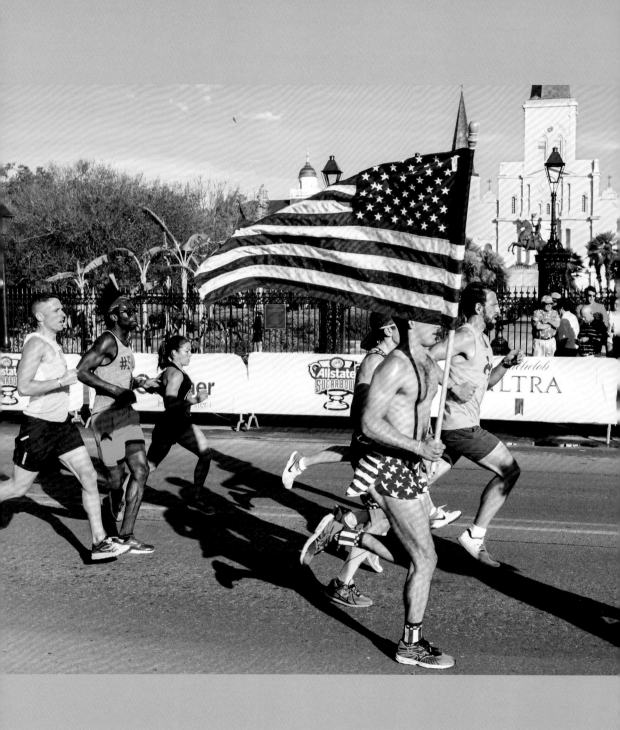

CRESCENT CITY CLASSIC

RECOMMENDED BY **Eric Stuart**

The Crescent City Classic has been called the original party race. Eric Stuart is happy to explain why. "For starters, we have what has to be the best post-race party anywhere, with the kind of food and entertainment you'd expect from New Orleans. Second, there's the open attitude the city has. With no open container laws, the party can extend onto the streets. Another aspect of the race that lends to its convivial atmosphere is the Classic's Everyman quality. You'll see a lot of average Joes out there walking the course, maybe as part of a New Year's resolution. You'll see people pushing strollers or pulling along a wagon with a keg of beer. [Such casual participants are in their own corral, or grouping.] Sometimes, people who've been having brunch or those who've been at the bars until the early morning will spill out and walk part of the course. It's a big social event in New Orleans. After Christmas, people begin talking about it—'What are you going to do for the Classic this year?' It always falls the Saturday before Easter, and people plan their weekend around it."

The first Crescent City Classic was run in 1979 and was the brainchild of a recent New Orleans émigré named Mac DeVaughn. Recognizing America's growing interest in running, Mac, a former banker, purchased a running shoe store. He came upon the idea of organizing a 10K to stimulate interest in the sport in a town that was inclined toward slightly more *sedentary* activities. Mac understood that a little star power could help put the nascent race on the map, and by calling in a few favors, he was able to persuade Frank Shorter—at that time, the biggest name in US racing—to run in the first race. Shorter bested the other 901 participants, and the Classic was established. Mac was able to continue to attract elite runners to New Orleans; in fact, in 1981, Michael Musyoki, a runner for the University of Texas at El Paso and native of Kenya,

OPPOSITE:
The Crescent City Classic— which weaves through the French Quarter, among other New Orleans neighborhoods— is a major social event every spring in the Big Easy.

DESTINATION

30

set a world record at the Classic, breaking the twenty-eight-minute mark. "By later in the 1980s, we had thirty-five thousand participants, making the Classic the biggest footrace in the world at the time," Eric continued. "Part of the appeal was certainly the laid-back atmosphere of New Orleans, but many high-caliber runners were drawn here because it's a very fast course. There aren't too many hills in the city. We had the fastest 10K time run in the last three years. But I would say that a majority of people don't worry too much about posting a great time. Of twenty-five thousand runners, I'd say that fifteen thousand are in costumes of some sort—lots of Easter bunnies, superheroes, figures of New Orleans history and acclaim. In 2016, there was one group that had constructed a *Back to the Future*–style DeLorean over a wagon and pulled it along the course . . . with a keg in the middle."

The course the Crescent City Classic takes has evolved since 1979 and is now in its fourth iteration. "The race used to begin in the French Quarter," Eric explained, "but as it evolved, the thinking went, 'Why rush through the French Quarter? Let's take our time.' Today, the race begins at the Superdome, goes through the central business district, and then passes Jackson Square, which signals your entry into the French Quarter. Running through the French Quarter, you'll pass Café Du Monde and the French Market before turning left on Esplanade Avenue, with its wonderful old mansions. You'll take Esplanade all the way down to Bayou St. John and the entrance to New Orleans City Park, America's second-largest park. You'll run most of the park up to Lelong Avenue and the finish line at the New Orleans Museum of Art. Most of the course is shaded, and at that time of the year—late March or early to mid-April—the temperature is perfect, around 55 or 60 degrees. From the finish line, you walk across the bridge to RaceFest."

RaceFest encompasses everything you'd expect from a party that follows New Orleans' most esteemed running race. "The twenty-five thousand Classic participants are joined by another twenty thousand partygoers," Eric described, "who can get in for a modest fee. All the great food you'd expect in New Orleans is available—jambalaya, red beans and rice, oysters, gumbo, and more. Beer (from sponsor Michelob Ultra) and Bloody Marys are flowing. The first band takes the stage at eight thirty A.M.; the next comes on at ten thirty A.M. We get the best New Orleans musicians to perform; past acts have included Big Sam's Funky Nation, Kermit Ruffins, and Rockin' Dopsie Jr. & the Zydeco Twisters. The park is really rocking. Most years, we have to push people out at one P.M. when RaceFest concludes."

RaceFest is not the only party associated with the Crescent City Classic. On the Thursday and Friday before the race, there's a free Health & Fitness Expo at the Hyatt Regency in downtown New Orleans. In addition to cooking and yoga demonstrations and exhibitions showcasing the latest in running and exercise equipment, there's lots of food and drink to be sampled.

The "Everyman" quality of the race that Eric mentioned is exemplified by a story he shared from the 2015 event. "It was about twelve fifteen or twelve thirty, and my team was beginning to take down the finish line because we figured everyone had finished," he recalled. "I looked down the course and saw this huge man making his way in our direction. He must have been four hundred pounds, but he was jogging, and he had three family members around him, offering encouragement. I was dumbstruck. It had taken him four hours to complete the course, but he was doing it. I imagine it was one of the great physical accomplishments in his life, and his family was there to share it with him."

ERIC STUART is the race director of the Allstate Sugar Bowl Crescent City Classic, a role he's held since 2012. He attended LSU on a track scholarship and was all-SEC seven times in cross-country, 800M, and distance relays. Eric worked for Hewlett-Packard for twenty-five years and took early retirement in 2012. He is an original member of the Greater New Orleans Sports Foundation and has helped produce three Super Bowls, four Final Fours, several National Championships, and the 1992 US Olympic Track & Field Trials. Eric has been married for thirty-eight years and has three kids and six grandkids.

If You Go

▶ **Getting There:** New Orleans is served by most major carriers.
▶ **Best Time to Visit:** The Crescent City Classic is held on the Saturday before Easter.
▶ **Race Information:** All details about the Classic, including entry information, can be found at the Crescent City Classic website (ccc10k.com).
▶ **Accommodations:** The Hyatt Regency New Orleans (504-561-1234; neworleans.regency.hyatt.com) is the official host hotel. The Crescent City Classic website lists other nearby lodging options.

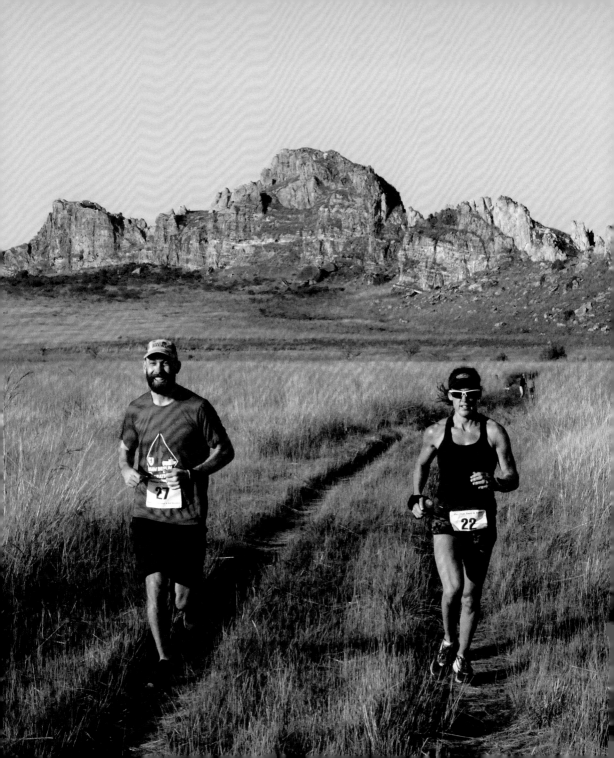

MADAGASCAR MARATHON

RECOMMENDED BY **Thom Gilligan**

Geologists believe that Madagascar—the world's fourth-largest island, roughly 250 miles southeast of Mozambique—has been separated from the continent of Africa for at least 150 million years—plenty of time for specialized ecosystems and many endemic species to evolve. Indeed, Madagascar has ten thousand animals and plants that are found nowhere else in the world . . . and scientists find new insects, reptiles, and plants almost every year. Madagascar—sometimes called the eighth continent—is not for the uninformed traveler. Schedule delays and itinerary changes are to be expected. Most roads have corroded asphalt and large potholes. Yet Madagascar offers attractions and adventures not found anywhere else. Some years ago, Thom Gilligan saw the opportunity to add a marathon to those sundry attractions.

"I was attending a Condé Nast event where various travel specialists were being honored," Thom began. "At one event where we were being wined and dined, a representative from Madagascar—Monique Rodriguez—introduced herself and suggested that I bring a group to Madagascar to run. I replied that I knew nothing of the island nation and perhaps should first come to visit. Arrangements were made, and I visited. I had a ten-day tour of the island and participated in a modest half marathon. In the course of the tour, I saw much of the country, often by four-wheel-drive vehicle, crossing rivers, driving through the forest and on horrid roads, visiting villages where people were afraid of cameras. Thanks to Monique, I learned a great deal quickly.

"Our slogan at Marathon Tours is 'Explore the seven continents one stride at a time.' We see running as a catalyst to get people to interesting places, and Madagascar certainly fit the bill. It was still so unexplored and pure; anthropologists still don't know where the Malagasy people came from—the South Pacific? Africa? India? There just aren't many tourists there.

OPPOSITE:
Running the
Madagascar
Marathon
provides an
excellent excuse
for visiting
a remarkable
country that's
been called
"the eighth
continent."

DESTINATION

31

In 2008, I brought a group of fifty-five runners over to run in the half marathon. It was primitively organized. I managed to rent an ATV and buy Cokes and bananas to support my group. Then we did a tour. The trip was successful, and I had many other people who were interested in going, but the event was canceled after 2008." Thom tried to organize a few other trips to Madagascar, but there were complications, and it kept getting pushed back. "I had to cancel a trip in 2013, and I'd get an email a month from clients wondering if there was going to be another," Thom continued. "Finally I went over again to see if I could organize a new race. I met a brother and sister who owned a hotel (Jardin du Roy) that was right on a trail that runs through Isalo National Park [in the southern part of Madagascar]. Better yet, the brother is an ultramarathoner. We created a course and advertised the race and sold out to one hundred people in three weeks."

The course that runners take through Isalo offers insights into both the natural and cultural wonders of Madagascar. "You run through a variety of habitats—some rolling grasslands, stands of palmlike trees, even a little rain forest area," Thom described. "At one point, you run past these stunning limestone formations called *tsingy*, which are believed to be 150 million years old. Later, you run down an old riverbed with fifteen-foot walls on either side. In the rain forest section, the trail crosses three or four creeks. The route also passes through three different villages. The people have almost nothing—no electricity, no cell phones, no running water. If they have a well or a pump to get water, it's considered a luxury. [According to the World Bank, Madagascar is one of the poorest countries in the world, with a per capita annual income of $260 in 2015.] They raise corn and use zebu (a breed of cattle) to plow their fields. Some of the villagers also keep rice paddies." One ray of economic hope in the Isalo region was the discovery of sapphires— some of the purest in the world—in the early 1990s.

"Of course, the local people can't afford the ten-dollar entry fee, but we plan to sponsor some runners on our next trip," Thom said. "The Malagasy like to run. They're not quite at the level of the East Africans, but they're good, and there are lots of running clubs. It's surprising to see so many people out running, considering it's such a poor country. You wonder how they can find the time and the food necessary to propel them along."

Thanks to the popularity of the DreamWorks animated film *Madagascar* and its two sequels, even the most indifferent naturalist will likely be able to identify Madagascar's signature mammal—the lemur. The lemur is a primate that can only be found on the island. They have been likened in appearance to a cross between a cat, a dog, and a squirrel, and in behavior, to monkeys . . . though they are a species unto themselves. At present, there are fifty-seven recognized taxa of lemurs, ranging in size from the tiny pygmy mouse lemur, which weighs less than an ounce, to the indri, which can reach twenty pounds. "We sometimes will come upon lemurs in Isalo National Park, but we're sure to encounter them in the rain forests near Antasibe, on the east coast," Thom added. "Here, we'll likely see indris, the largest species of lemur, which refuse to eat when held in captivity and die. At a spot called Lemur Island, we'll see another species of lemur, sifaka. They are so humanlike, with soft little hands. They even look at you like a person. "The Malagasy believe that mankind evolved from lemurs."

THOM GILLIGAN founded Marathon Tours & Travel in 1979 and still acts as CEO. Named the top specialist in running-related travel by *Condé Nast Traveler* magazine nine times, he has also been featured in *Runner's World*, on the front page of the *Wall Street Journal*, and on the cover of *Travel Agent* magazine. Thom personally leads groups to marathons in Bermuda, France's Bordeaux region, and more, including Antarctica, where he is the race director and expedition leader for the Antarctica Marathon. A former president of the Greater Boston Track Club, Thom has run sixty-two marathons around the world, with a personal best of 2:30:42. An avid golfer, he holds a four handicap and admits that he is hopelessly addicted.

If You Go

▶ **Getting There:** Several carriers provide service to Madagascar, including Air France (800-237-2747; airfrance.com) and South African Airways (954-769-5000; flysaa.com). Marathon Tours & Travel can arrange air bookings at group rates and manages all internal flights for guests.

▶ **Best Time to Visit:** The Madagascar Marathon is held in mid-June.

▶ **Race Information:** Marathon Tours & Travel (617-242-7845; marathontours.com) created the event and organizes both the race and accompanying tours of Madagascar.

▶ **Accommodations:** Lodging for the Madagascar Marathon (and tours) is coordinated by Marathon Tours & Travel. This includes a stay at Jardin du Roy (lejardinduroy.com).

DESTINATION

31

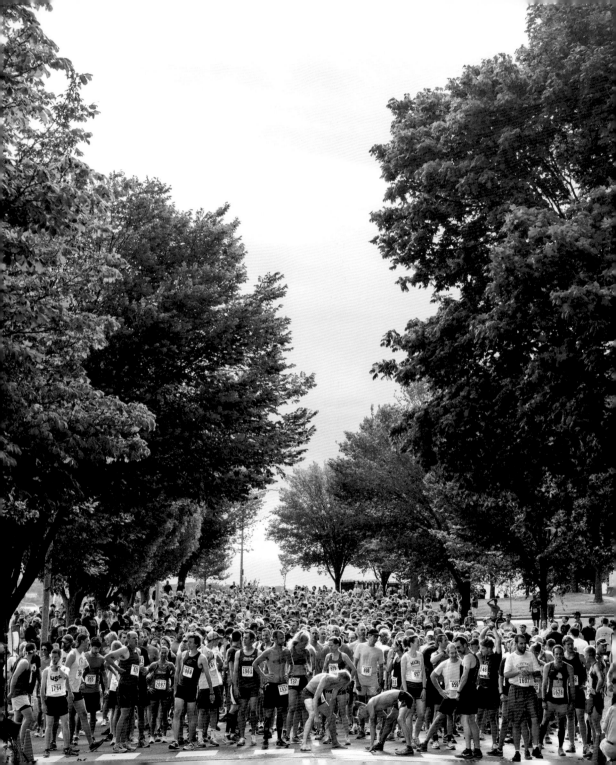

TRAIL TO ALE 10K

RECOMMENDED BY **Chris Harmon**

Portland—the picturesque and diminutive city (population around seventy thousand) that rests two hours north of Boston along Maine's Casco Bay—brings many of Maine's best facets together in one place. Here, the sandy beaches that characterize the southern part of the Pine Tree State's shoreline meet the rock-ribbed, cove-laden coast that's conjured up by the phrase "Downeast Maine." Portland has a thriving restaurant and music scene that belies its modest population. On a summer Saturday night, the city's cobblestoned Old Port neighborhood is swinging with live rock and jazz from pubs resting on pilings over the harbor.

OPPOSITE: Trail to Ale celebrates two of Portland's passions: green space and beer.

A major part of Portland's appeal is its far sighted mission to protect urban land from overdevelopment; the city boasts 721 acres of green space, including trails, gardens, athletic fields, and more. This commitment to green space is celebrated with the Trail to Ale 10K—an event that combines bay vistas, pizza, and locally crafted beer.

"I first heard about the Trail to Ale from my dad, who coaches cross-country at a local high school," Chris Harmon began. "I was attending my first year in law school at the time in Portland and helping him coach, and I thought it was a great idea. The first year I ran, I cramped up a bit, thanks to my celiac disease—which I didn't realize that I had at the time. Even though the race didn't go as well for me as it might have, I loved the event. It really brings the community together and combines a few of my loves—the local breweries and Portland Trails, which is a great organization."

Portland Trails is a nonprofit that was formed in 1990 to advocate for a connected trail system in the city limits. What began as an all-volunteer organization has grown to six employees, more than one thousand members, and nearly one thousand volunteers, including seven hundred volunteers devoting some six thousand hours to trail maintenance.

DESTINATION

32

Technically, Portland Trails operates as a land trust; though the organization owns more than one hundred acres of land, much of the access to green space they've secured is in the form of easements. Today, the trail network reaches within half a mile of every residence in Portland, spans four communities, and is used by joggers, bicyclists, and people just looking for a safe and pleasant path from point A to point B. (In addition to maintaining its trail network, Portland Trails engages in placemaking—which Project for Public Spaces defines as "a collaborative process by which we can shape our public realm in order to maximize shared value"—and school ground greening, which helps engage students with natural surroundings close to their schools.)

Two of the most popular trails in the system—which play a pivotal role in the Trail to Ale event—are Back Cove and the Eastern Promenade. Back Cove Trail circles its eponymous body of water (or mud flats at low tide) for 3.6 miles, with great views of Portland's skyline as one looks to the east. "Back Cove might be Maine's most popular running route," Chris continued. "I try to incorporate it into every run. It's six feet wide, packed gravel with mile markers and workout stops. I grew up running it with my family." Back Cove connects to the Eastern Promenade, which is built along an old narrow-gauge rail corridor with resplendent views of Portland Harbor and the ocean beyond. "From the Eastern Promenade, you look out on Mackworth Island and Hog Island, which has an old Civil War–era fort, as well as other islands in the distance," Chris added. "There's a beautiful park here; it's the first place that I take visitors from out of town."

The evolution of Portland's trail system coincided with the dawn of its craft brewing scene, which can be traced to 1986, when David Geary and his wife, Karen, poured the first pints of Geary's Pale Ale. Geary was followed a few years later (in 1994) by Shipyard, which has grown to be one of America's larger craft breweries, shipping their flagship Export Ale to all fifty states; and Allagash Brewing, which began selling beer in 1995 and has built a national reputation with its Belgian-inspired ales, particularly Allagash White. As of this writing, Portland is home to a dozen small breweries, with a smattering of other operations to the north and south.

The Trail to Ale is run in mid-September. Chris described the course: "The race begins up on a hill, just a bit south of the Eastern Promenade, on the Bayside Trail. This leads downhill on the outskirts of downtown until it connects with the Back Cove Trail. After the Back Cove, you hit the first little uphill as you go past Tukey's Bridge; here, you might smell baked beans, as the plant that makes B&M Baked Beans is across the bridge. Past the bridge, you come onto the Eastern Promenade. Mackworth Island is to your left as you approach the race's end near the public boat launch.

"Just above the boat launch at a park overlooking the water, the main brewing sponsor—Shipyard—has ale flowing. There's also great local pizza [from Portland Pie Company]. Because I have celiac disease, I can't partake much of the pizza and beer. But my fiancée can. [Fortunately for Chris, Shipyard owns Capt'n Eli's, a gourmet soda company, and their product is also flowing!] There's a fun dance party with a DJ after the race, free yoga and massages, a great community of runners, and a tremendous water view. It all makes this race very special . . . that, and the fact that this was also the first race that my fiancée and I ran together when we started dating. Now we try to run it together every year."

CHRIS HARMON attended the University of Maine, earning the Eugene Mawhinney Award for graduating as the valedictorian in his major, political science. He also graduated from the University of Maine School of Law, earned a spot on the editorial board of the Maine Law Review, and served as president of the student body. Chris is one of Maine's most accomplished amateur runners, having placed second in the Maine Marathon, twenty-fifth overall in the Beach to Beacon, and first in the Trail to Ale 10K. His legal practice (with Terry Garmey and Associates) focuses on multi-district litigation, products liability, and slip and fall cases.

DESTINATION 32

If You Go

► **Getting There:** Portland is served by many carriers, including Delta (800-221-1212; delta.com) and United (800-864-8331; united.com).

► **Best Time to Visit:** The Trail to Ale event is held in mid-September. You can count on fairly good running weather between mid-May and mid-October.

► **Race Information:** Details about the race, including registration information, are available at trails.org/events/races/trail-to-ale. The Portland Trails site (trails.org) also details the many trail options around Portland.

► **Accommodations:** Visit Portland (207-772-5800; visitportland.com) lists accommodations in the city.

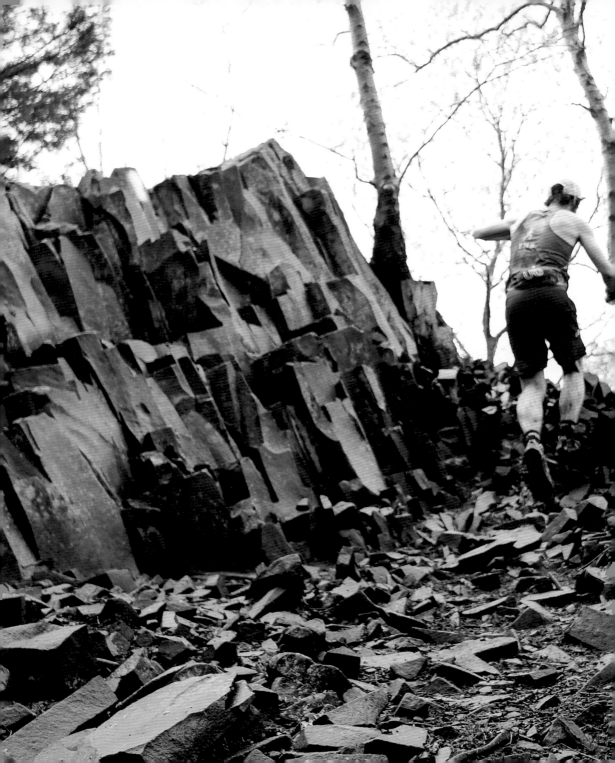

SEVEN SISTERS TRAIL RACE

RECOMMENDED BY **Brian Rusiecki**

It was cycling that initially brought Brian Rusiecki to trail running and the Seven Sisters Trail. "I was a competitive cyclist through high school and college," he began, "but after a while, I got burnt out. A lot of the participants were very competitive; there was so much fancy gear. I realized that I just wasn't enjoying it anymore. Even though it was getting me outside, there were cars buzzing by, which took away from the experience. And I was on a machine that was kind of uncomfortable. I realized I wanted to go for a hike, maybe jog some. I put two and two together and realized that trail running satisfied a lot of these desires. I realized I was pretty good at handling the off-camber terrain. I wouldn't get super tired after all the years of cycling, and I wouldn't fall down. And there was no goofy spandex and other equipment. Just grab your shoes and off you go.

"Seven Sisters was a local trail. In the past, I used to hike it, run down some of the hills. I'd go out there and run on the weekend to stay fit for biking. I didn't know people did trail running for sport."

This swath of Massachusetts—sometimes called the Pioneer Valley—remains mostly idyllic, despite its relative proximity to the hustle and bustle of Boston (less than two hours to the east). Shaped in part by the Connecticut River, it's a land of tidy organic farms (and farm-to-table restaurants), prestigious prep schools, potters and other artisans, singer-songwriters, and assorted urban émigrés from Manhattan and beyond. The term Seven Sisters references a ridgeline between Mount Holyoke and Mount Hitchcock that's part of the larger Holyoke Range. While the "knobs" of the ridge go no higher than 945 feet, they rise and fall abruptly, making this section of the Metacomet-Monadnock (or "M-M") Trail one of New England's most rigorous trail-running courses.

OPPOSITE:
Though none of
the mountains on
the Seven Sisters
Trail Race course
exceed one
thousand feet,
the ups and
downs can
be punishing.

DESTINATION

33

While some self-avowed road runners will run trails and vice versa, almost all would agree that they are different endeavors that both involve running. The International Trail Running Association defines trail running as follows:

> Trail running is a pedestrian race open to all, in a natural environment (mountain, desert, forest, plain . . .) with minimal possible paved or asphalt road (which should not exceed 20 percent of the total course). The terrain can vary (dirt road, forest trail, single track . . .) and the route must be properly marked. The race is ideally—but not necessarily—in self-sufficiency or semi-self-sufficiency, and is held in the respect for sporting ethics, loyalty, solidarity, and the environment.

Whereas the birth of twentieth-century trail running can be traced to Marin County's Dipsea in 1905 (or, if you prefer ultra events, the Western States® 100-Mile Endurance Run in 1974), *Trail Run* magazine traces the first recorded trail run to 1040 in Scotland, where "King Malcolm Canmore organized a race in Braemar, reputedly to find a swift messenger." Brian simply summed up two of the main differences between road and trail running: "There's a lot of stuff in your way, and it can be very steep, up and down. You have to keep focused to keep from falling."

The course for the Seven Sisters is twelve miles, out and back, on a single-track trail. "It's truly single track, really narrow," Brian continued. "In the summer the foliage gets thick, and you're going through a tunnel of green. Even though the trail gets traffic, it's tight in there. In the winter, you can see much better. I run the trail a lot; honestly, I don't know if there's anyone who runs it more than I do. But after every run, I say to myself, 'That was hard.' It never seems easy. But at the same time, you're never bored. There are so many ups and downs, you kind of lose track of whether you're on one of the hills or not . . . though at the high points, you have some nice lookouts over the five colleges, the Connecticut River, and farmland. There are more than seven hills, that's for sure. I try to run them all—they're very jagged and very steep. Going up, your heart rate gets jacked, as if you're doing a bunch of intervals. If you go out for a two-hour road run, you can dictate your heart rate. When you go on the Seven Sisters and try to run everything, your heart rate is all over."

The Seven Sisters Trail Race grew from an informal event inaugurated by two local runners, Fred Pilon and Peter Crisci, in the late 1980s. There was pushback from the Forest Service, but once a local land trust called Friends of the Holyoke Range stepped in, helping to reimagine the event as a fund-raiser for the organization, the restrictions were lifted. The first official race was run in 1991. Today the race, which happens in early May, attracts up to six hundred runners; nearly $100,000 has been raised for the organization.

"The Seven Sisters was the first race I ran when I felt, wow, I did pretty good," Brian recalled. "Some of the guys competing were among the best in the area. It was my first big win. And that run, I also got a chance to get to know better the woman who's now my wife. She won too. That started our bond."

BRIAN RUSIECKI transitioned from cycling to trail running due to his envy of the simplicity and solitude of the sport. He went from never running to running his first fifty-miler within a year and never looked back. With his mentality that "a two-hour run is good, so four hours must be better," Brian has racked up the miles and the races, completing about one hundred ultras in ten years. He's won many races up and down the East Coast, including the Vermont 100 (three times, breaking the course record in 2014), the Vermont 50 (four times), the Massanutten 100 (two times), the Hellgate 100K, and the Mountain Masochist (two times), and has been ranked one of the top ten ultra-runners in North America for the last five years. Brian's feet hardly ever touch pavement while he is accumulating his non-racing miles around his home in Western Massachusetts. He is sponsored by Patagonia, HOKA ONE ONE, and Drymax.

DESTINATION

33

If You Go

▶ **Getting There:** The closest jetport to Amherst is in Hartford, Connecticut, which is served by many carriers, including Delta (800-221-1212; delta.com) and United (800-864-8331; united.com).

▶ **Best Time to Visit:** The Seven Sisters Trail Run occurs in early May. Early fall is also a wonderful time to be in Western Massachusetts.

▶ **Race Information:** Details on the race (including registration information) and the trail reside at 7sisterstrailrace.com.

▶ **Accommodations:** The Amherst Area Chamber of Commerce (413-253-0700; amherst area.com) lists lodging options in the region.

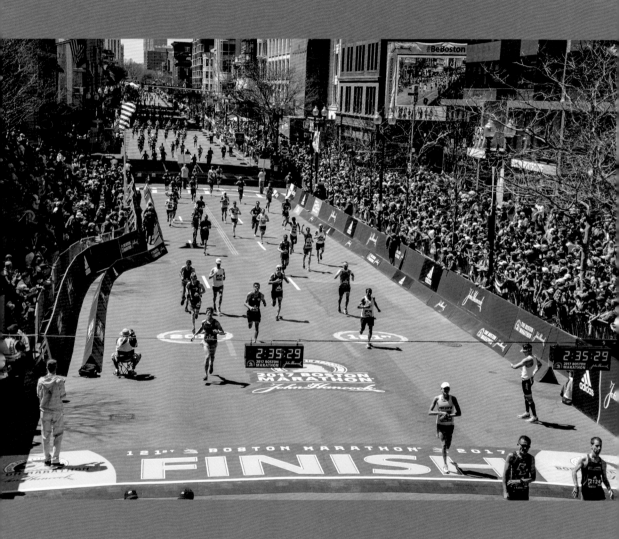

BOSTON MARATHON

RECOMMENDED BY **Dave McGillivray**

The course has changed little since the race was first run in 1897. It's a badge of honor to simply qualify for it. It's a chance to run on the hallowed ground that the best runners in the world have battled on for the last century.

For Dave McGillivray, the Boston Marathon has been a labor of love for much of his life. "I've done it for forty-four years in a row; it's in my DNA," he began. "I didn't create the race, but as race director, I'm a caretaker for a period of time . . . though I'm really more a conductor than a director, as we have such a well-oiled, experienced team in place. I hope to pass it on to the next guy or gal without messing it up. The Boston Marathon is a magnet that draws the best runners from around the world; it's not the Olympics, but it's close. There are all those iconic spots along the route—Wellesley College, Heartbreak Hill, the Citgo sign. Once you see that sign and can smell the ocean, nothing can stop you. Some [finishes] might not be as pretty as others, but odds are you'll get there. Ninety-nine percent do."

Dave clearly recalls his first crack at the marathon. "I was seventeen and decided I wanted to do the race. But I was too young. I jumped in anyway. Before I started, I called up my grandfather, who lived near the course, and he said he would meet me at Coolidge Corner, mile twenty-four. I got as far as the hills in Newton and down I went; I'd never gone farther than eleven miles before. I was taken to Newton-Wellesley Hospital by ambulance. I called my grandfather and he asked, 'Where have you been?' I told him what happened and apologized for failing. He said, 'You didn't fail; you learned. You can't go and set reckless goals. If you train hard, I'll be there for you next year.' Unfortunately, he died. I entered the next year (legally) and was really fit, but got sick the day before. My parents didn't want me to run, but I did anyway. I got as far as Newton and found myself

OPPOSITE:
A chance to participate in— and finish— the Boston Marathon is a must on any serious runner's bucket list.

DESTINATION

34

155

doing the survivor shuffle. I was ready to drop out at mile 21.5. I figured it was not meant to be—I shouldn't be a marathoner. I looked around behind me and saw the cemetery where my grandfather lay. He said he'd be there, and he was. I got up and finished for Grandpa—my time was 4.5 hours."

When asked about the most memorable stretches of the route, Dave paused. "Every part of the course has significance," he started. "Take the three hills in Newton after mile 17.5. Some people think the first is Heartbreak. Then the second. It's the third. The Evergreen Cemetery stretch between Boston College and Cleveland Circle—the 'haunted mile'—is also tough. When you come out of Boston College, the crowds are ten deep, but then suddenly you're in a void, with the cemetery on the right and the trolley line on the left. Many runners lose it here. You have to hang on until you get to Beacon Street. That gets people going. Running by Fenway Park at mile twenty-five is exciting; the park is as old and iconic as the race. We've worked it out with the Red Sox so that runners can come back to Fenway for a post-race party on the field."

So many powerful, inspiring tales have sprung from the Boston Marathon over the years . . . and that's without even mentioning the bravery and resilience of the runners who survived the 2013 bombing and returned to run again. One story from Dave's thirty years as race director that has stuck with him is a bit smaller, perhaps, but no less a tribute to the power of sportsmanship and the human spirit. "Some years back, I had a call from a woman named Katie. She wanted to come by the office to chat. She rolled in in a wheelchair and went into our conference room. When I came in, my jaw dropped. She had dwarfism and was twenty-six inches tall. 'I have a question, Mr. McGillivray. Can I run in the marathon?' I paused for a moment and then said, 'Yes, you can.' But then she said she had a caveat: that her marathon is 26.2 feet.

"As race day grew closer, she trained like crazy in her walker. When the marathon came, I cordoned off a section 26.2 feet from the starting line. All the best runners in the world were there, everyone screaming. She finished in 7.5 minutes. When she crossed her finish line, I gave her a medal and a laurel wreath. Then the official race began.

"Since I became involved in [organizing] the race twenty-nine years ago, I haven't been able to run with everyone else. That first year I couldn't run, I was there at the finish line, elated for all the finishers but full of self-pity for me. Then I had an idea. I asked a state trooper if he would take me to the start. I took off from the start line at eight P.M. and finished dead last. I've been the last finisher twenty-nine years in a row, since 1988. Generally, it's just me and a few friends at the finish line.

"That night, as I'm coming in at eleven o'clock, I can see one person in the distance. As I get closer, I can see that it's Katie. When I crossed the finish line, she put a medal that she made and a laurel wreath that she made around my neck. She said, 'Ha, I beat ya!' Katie died a few years later, and I sense that she knew she didn't have much time left when she first came to see me. She wanted one opportunity, and we gave her that."

DAVE MCGILLIVRAY has been the race director of the Boston Marathon since 1988 and has completed the race forty-five consecutive years . . . and 145 marathons overall. He is the owner and president of Dave McGillivray Sports Enterprises Inc. (DMSE), which since 1982 has produced or consulted on almost one thousand mass-participatory athletic events nationally and internationally. Dave first received attention in 1978 when he ran a total of 3,452 miles in eighty days to raise money for the Jimmy Fund of Boston. Many millions of dollars have been raised for charity both through his personal efforts and by events DMSE has managed. For his inspiring work, Dave has been recognized with many honors, including *Competitor* magazine's Lifetime Achievement Award in 2000; induction into the Running USA Hall of Champions in January of 2005; and the Jimmy Award, which honors celebrities who have committed themselves to the mission of the Dana-Farber Cancer Institute and the Jimmy Fund. He is a much sought-after motivational speaker. Learn more about his many accomplishments at dmsesports.com.

If You Go

► **Getting There:** Boston is served by most major carriers.
► **Best Time to Visit:** The Boston Marathon is held on Patriots' Day, which falls on the third Monday in April.
► **Race Information:** The Boston Marathon has stringent entry requirements, including a qualifying time at a recognized marathon. Details about entry and other aspects of the race can be found at the Boston Athletic Association website (baa.org).
► **Accommodations:** The Greater Boston Convention & Visitors Bureau (888-SEE-BOSTON; bostonusa.com) lists lodging options throughout the city.

DESTINATION

34

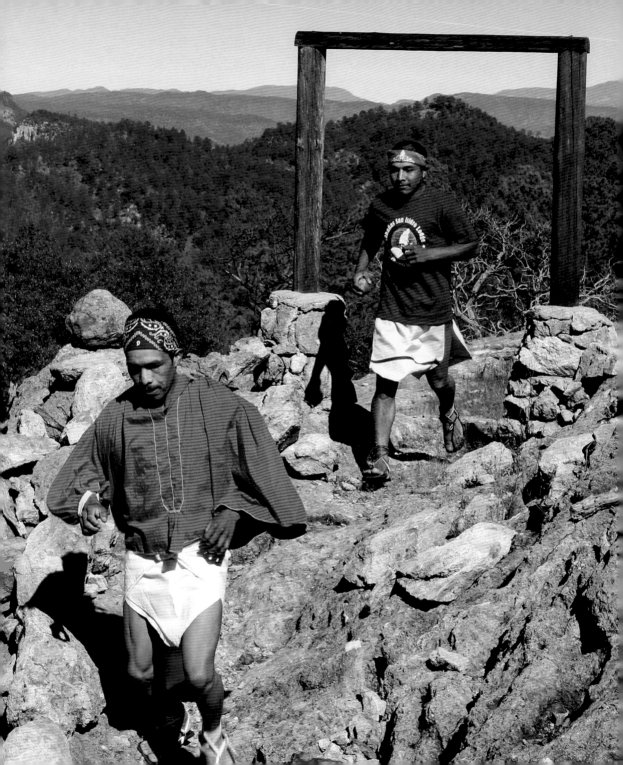

COPPER CANYON

RECOMMENDED BY **Dave Hensleigh**

Long before gringos ever considered running without shoes or seeking the wisdom of the Rarámuri (often called the Tarahumara) people, Dave Hensleigh had set his sights on Mexico's Copper Canyon. "One of my brothers had made the trip years back," Dave recalled, "and his stories of the native people and the canyons had always been in the back of my head. When I first saw Copper Canyon, I was amazed at its ruggedness. It was this ruggedness, at least in part, that helped the Rarámuri resist the Spanish conquistadores, because the Spanish couldn't reach them as they fled deeper into the canyon country. On one of my early trips, I hiked to the bottom of the canyon and back up in a day. I was incredibly spent. The next day, at a tiny grocery store in one of the villages, I saw a kid with a sack of oranges. I asked where he'd gotten them, and he said at the bottom of the canyon . . . that morning! This spoke to the incredible endurance and strength of these shy, somewhat reclusive people. I was fascinated."

The name Copper Canyon—*Barranca del Cobre* in Spanish—is often used to refer to a series of six immense gorges that cut through the Sierra Madre Occidental in the state of Chihuahua in northwestern Mexico. Overall, Copper Canyon is four times the size of Arizona's Grand Canyon, and four of the gorges are deeper by as much as one thousand feet. Though the Spanish found silver here, copper was never discovered; rather, the formation takes its name from the copper-colored lichen that grows on many of the canyon walls. The region boasts a tremendous diversity of ecosystems given its dramatic range in elevation, and this has attracted outdoor recreationists from the United States and beyond.

Few recent books have sparked as many conversations in the running community as Christopher McDougall's *Born to Run*, an exploration of the Rarámuri and their incredible running ability, Copper Canyon, and the very nature of running. In an interview with

OPPOSITE: The Rarámuri run in simple huaraches, most of which are made from recycled tires.

DESTINATION

35

Amazon.com, McDougall explained how his time in Copper Canyon changed his quest:

> It was this: Everything I'd been taught about running was wrong. We treat running in the modern world the same way we treat childbirth—it's going to hurt, and requires special exercises and equipment, and the best you can hope for is to get it over with quickly with minimal damage. Then I meet the Tarahumara, and they're having a blast. They remember what it's like to love running, and it lets them blaze through the canyons like dolphins rocketing through waves. For them, running isn't work. It isn't a punishment for eating. It's fine art, like it was for our ancestors.

Thanks in part to McDougall's book, Copper Canyon has begun appearing on more runners' bucket lists than ever before. A more commercial legacy of *Born to Run*, however, has been the birth of minimalist running shoes, such as the toe shoe. The Rarámuri run with simple sandals called huaraches, which promote a more natural gait while offering protection from sharp rocks and other detritus. Most have soles made from recycled tires.

"I had been leading cultural tours to the Copper Canyon region for several years, and it was about the time that *Born to Run* came out that I started thinking about a running-oriented tour," Dave continued. "During one visit, I met with Gustavo Lozano, who had laid out the original Caballo Blanco Ultramarathon course. He told me that some of the young runners wanted to come and compete in America. I asked him, 'Where does Miguel Lara [who had won the Caballo Blanco] live?' We set off one morning through gullies and over a ridge, and eventually came to a little cabin. There was a young man wearing cowboy boots and a baseball cap, shelling beans—it was Miguel. I asked if he could show me how he ran. He took off up a ridge, feet a little wider apart, staying close to the ground. I asked if he could run down, and he did. I thought right then that I was going to do something with these guys." One of the things Dave did with Miguel, Arnulfo Quimare, and other great Rarámuri runners was bring them to the United States to compete in a number of races. He has also brought American runners to Copper Canyon to run with the Rarámuri. "When we do a running trip, it's not me taking guests on a trail I heard about from the guys," Dave added. "It's one of the locals who is guiding you."

Excursions to run the trails of Copper Canyon with the Rarámuri are customized to meet a small group's desires. "Some people like a chance to take the famous Chihuahua al Pacifico Railroad and do some running at stops along the way," Dave explained. "I've also had some serious ultra-runners who didn't care about the train; they wanted to get in twenty or thirty miles a day. For this kind of group, I like to go directly to San Isidro Lodge. "It's run by some brothers who have nice little cabins and even a sweat lodge. It's a tremendous place to run from, as there are a variety of trails that depart from here. The guides can take you on the most rigorous terrain or more modest options. If a group desires to participate in one of the big ultra events like the Caballo Blanco in early March, that can be arranged too. The food is a special part of the experience. It's hearty ranch fare, not fancy at all, but delicious. There's also a chance to sample the local drink. *Lechuguilla* is the strong spirit. There's also a corn beer, *tesguino*."

There is a concept called *korima* that the Rarámuri hold dear—it connotes "what I have, you have." For Dave, a chance to experience this warmth is the main reason to visit Copper Canyon. "Copper Canyon takes your soul away; it's so spectacular, so vast, and so quiet. As you're running, you have to take it in. But what's lodged in my heart is a memory of the connection I've made with the people."

DAVE HENSLEIGH has been leading guests on trips to Mexico for more than thirty years. He started Authentic Copper Canyon to give curious travelers a vivid experience in the true life of the region and its people. A former pastor and longtime runner, Dave is ever in quest of his next personal record.

If You Go

▶ **Getting There:** Many visitors will fly into Chihuahua City or Mexico City. Chihuahua is served by a number of carriers, including Aeromexico (800-237-6639; aeromexico.com).

▶ **Best Time to Visit:** September through April sees cooler and less humid conditions in the canyon. Runners interested in the Caballo Blanco should visit in March.

▶ **Tour Information:** Dave Hensleigh's Authentic Copper Canyon (217-369-9897; authenticcoppercanyon.com) leads small, customized trips to the region and can arrange Rarámuri running guides.

▶ **Accommodations:** For solo travelers, there are a range of options in the towns along the Chihuahua al Pacifico Railroad line. Dave recommends San Isidro Lodge (+52 6354565257; coppercanyonamigos.com).

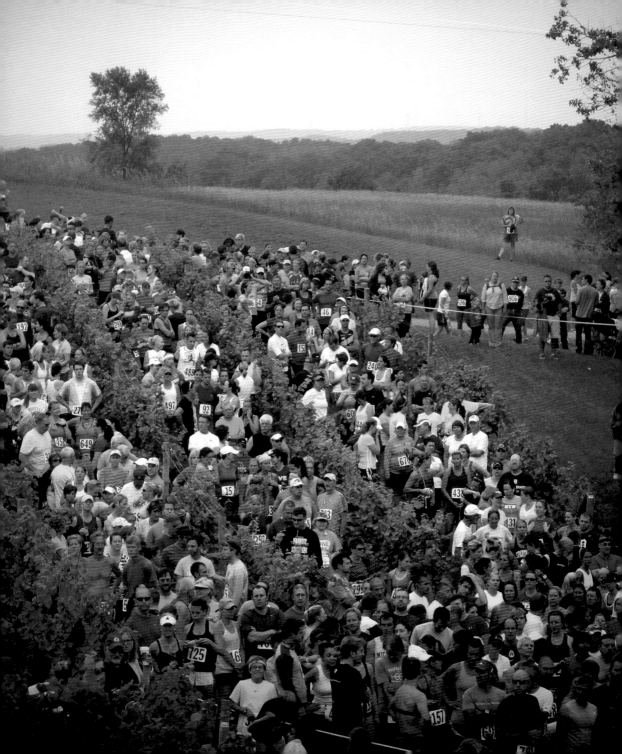

HARVEST STOMPEDE

RECOMMENDED BY **Rick Coates**

Traverse City sits at the mouth of Grand Traverse Bay, an inlet of Lake Michigan located toward the top of Michigan's Lower Peninsula. The deep woods and many lakes of the surrounding north country region have made Traverse City a four-season resort, popular with golfers, boaters, bicyclists, cross-country skiers, anglers, and those happy just to sit on the many white-sand beaches . . . at least in the summertime. Traverse City has long been known as America's cherry capital, producing more than 70 percent of the tart cherries grown in the United States. The region—particularly the Leelanau and Old Mission Peninsulas that jut out from Traverse City into Grand Traverse Bay—has emerged in the last few decades as a significant wine-producing region, creating Riesling, Chardonnay, Pinot Grigio, and Gewürztraminer as well as ice wines.

What better to promote a burgeoning wine region than a great race?

"One day in the late nineties, I was approached by the folks at Black Star Farms—one of the more established wineries on the Leelanau Peninsula—because they wanted to establish a wine trail to help market their product," Rick Coates recalled. "The owner of Black Star had been to the Finger Lakes region and wanted to replicate what they had. I went to a meeting, and before I knew it, I was running the program. I tried to assemble events along the trail based loosely on what had been done in New York, with our own northern Michigan spin. Tony Ciccone, who owns Ciccone Vineyard and Winery (and happens to be the father of an artist who goes by the name of Madonna), told me that one of his former employees was a runner, and thought it would be great to have a run through the vineyard. I looked into it, and he was right—there was potential for a really cool trail run. The first Harvest Stompede was held in 2001 and was a seven-mile run. It came off very well. There were a lot of people participating in the wine trail part of the

OPPOSITE:
Northern
Michigan's
Leelanau
Peninsula is
emerging as a
leading wine-
growing region—
and the Harvest
Stompede routes
a 10K through
one of its
vineyards.

DESTINATION

36

event who weren't competitive runners but wanted to participate, even if it meant walking. So we ended up adding a 5K run and a 5K walk. For a time, the 5K was called the Stinger. There was a mud wasp nest along the trail, and someone ran over it. More than fifty people got stung—we put a bee on the race T-shirt."

Given the extreme cold that visits northern Michigan in the wintertime, the Leelanau Peninsula's increasing popularity as a wine-making region may come as a surprise to many. Yet the lake effect—from Lake Michigan to the west and Grand Traverse Bay to the east—has a moderating effect on temperatures. The downdraft that's created also helps, delaying early blossoms and early frosts, and delivering ample snow to protect the vines from extreme cold snaps. In the early 1980s, there were only four wineries in the region— Boskydel Vineyard, Leelanau Wine Cellars, Good Harbor Vineyards, and L. Mawby Vineyards. Today, there are twenty-five wineries on the peninsula, and the Stompede is one of the year's biggest tasting events—a self-guided tour where visitors can enjoy a wine and food pairing at their choice of twenty-three participating vineyards. "When our wines first became noticed, there were lots of comparisons to California wines," Rick continued. "People would say, 'These aren't California reds.' No, they're Michigan reds. But when California began producing wines, people were comparing them to French wines. It's natural to make such comparisons. When the race started to bring in people from out of state, runners who hadn't come primarily for the wine were tasting and saying that some of our varietals were every bit as good as some coming from Europe, Australia, and even California. That was an exciting and gratifying time to be here."

The race kicks off at a leisurely nine A.M. at the Ciccone Vineyard and follows trails through Ciccone and adjoining land before returning to Ciccone for the conclusion. "The trails run right through the grapes, which are very ripe, as it's harvest time," Rick added. "You navigate some hills along the way, and there are some great views of Grand Traverse Bay and the peninsula beyond. To me, the Stompede combines elements of a serious race and a fun run. Some trail runners come here and take it very seriously, but for others, this may be one of their few runs of the year." The stomping area after the finish line certainly is a nod to the fun side of things. "Nate Rousse [race director] and Tony Ciccone thought we should have something at the end that people could jump into to celebrate the harvest—a vat full of grapes that people could stomp on. I said, 'Let's do it.' Finishers have the option of doing some stomping, but you don't have to . . . though onlookers are certainly cheering you on to get your feet wet."

Once the running is done, it's time for the tasting to begin. "There's something for everyone on the Leelanau," Rick opined. "There's the 'wow' factor of great views, elegant tasting rooms, and intimate tastings with winery owners. Chateau Fontaine, which is on the other side of the peninsula, brings all the elements together—exceptional wines and a wonderful tasting room with very engaging owners. L. Mawby is the sparkling wine guru of the Midwest. Black Star Farms has a fine restaurant on-site and offers some of the most creative pairings."

If you're more a fan of the hops than the grapes, take heart: Traverse City has more than a dozen craft breweries.

RICK COATES is a writer whose work has appeared in more than three hundred publications, along with a few books over the past thirty-eight years. His writing focuses on food and drink, culture, leisure, and celebrities. Rick lives in Traverse City, Michigan, with his wife and two children. When not writing he is often dining, drinking, golfing, and fly-fishing with rock stars and celebrity chefs.

If You Go

▶ **Getting There:** Traverse City is served by several carriers, including American Eagle (800-433-7300; aa.com) and Delta (800-221-1212; delta.com).
▶ **Best Time to Visit:** The Harvest Stompede is held the second weekend in September, a lovely time to visit northern Michigan.
▶ **Race Information:** Details about the Harvest Stompede, including registration information, are provided by the Leelanau Peninsula Wine Trail (231-642-5550; lpwines.com).
▶ **Accommodations:** Several wineries offer packages for the Stompede weekend, including Black Star Farms (231-944-1251; blackstarfarms.com) and Fairfield Inn and Suites, Traverse City (231-922-7900). Traverse City Tourism (800-872-8377; traversecity.com) lists other options.

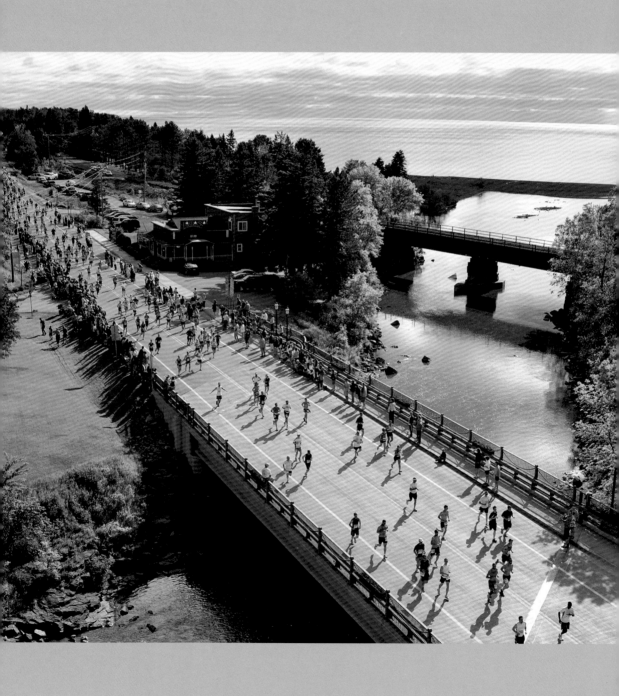

GRANDMA'S MARATHON

RECOMMENDED BY **Kate Kucinski**

There's a quote from Mark Twain—considered apocryphal by some—that goes: "The coldest winter I ever spent was a summer in Duluth." You'll have a chance to see for yourself when you compete in Grandma's Marathon, held in mid-June each year along the shores of Lake Superior.

"In some cities when there's a marathon going on, the average citizen might not be aware of it," Kate Kucinski began. "But in Duluth, Grandma's Marathon is a big deal. Grandma's tries to make every runner feel like a celebrity. June is a great time for a marathon, as our weather tends to be cool, and there's a nice breeze with a little fog blowing in off the lake—perfect conditions for running. It's the kickoff for our summer, and Duluth gets great community participation—more than six thousand volunteers, and many more spectators. It's part of the social calendar for many people. People in Duluth really come out—there are community bands, cheerleaders, kids with signs urging runners on. In 2016, there were runners from all fifty states and thirty-nine countries, more than eighteen thousand in the marathon and another three thousand in the half marathon and 5K. The cool weather and a fast course make Grandma's a favorite for people trying to qualify for the Boston Marathon. It makes residents of the region proud to look at the list of the nation's biggest marathons and find little Duluth there among the greats."

Duluth sits at the far southwestern corner of Lake Superior, the largest of the five Great Lakes and one of the largest lakes in the world. It grew to prominence as a port city; at one point in the early 1900s, Duluth handled more tonnage than New York, and it remains the biggest inland harbor in the world. In the latter half of the twentieth century, its fortunes as a port and steel producer waned. But city leaders, recognizing the potential of the waterfront (and seeing the success that cities like Boston, Baltimore, and Toronto

OPPOSITE: Grandma's Marathon (which takes its name from a local restaurant) takes runners along Lake Superior before concluding in Duluth.

DESTINATION

37

167

had experienced with their port revitalizations), set to work. Today, Duluth boasts the Lakewalk, Great Lakes Aquarium, Canal Park, and Duluth Entertainment Convention Center, among other attractions, and has enjoyed success drawing tourists and conventioneers. (The port is still active as well.) As for the Twain comment: US Climate Data reports an average high of 76 degrees in Duluth in July, though conditions at the lake do tend to be *a bit cooler*.

The genesis of Grandma's Marathon dates back to before the reimagining of Duluth, to 1976—and there were no actual grandmothers involved. "There was a running club in Duluth called the North Shore Striders," Kate continued. "They had put on some races in the area, and they used to do training runs along the lake from Two Harbors to Duluth on a route very similar to the one now used for the marathon. They decided that they should take the route and make it an official marathon event. One of the club members, Scott Keenan, worked at Grandma's Saloon and Grill, at that time a brand-new restaurant in Duluth. The Striders needed $650 to conduct the event, and he went to Grandma's after being turned down by a number of other potential sponsors. They agreed to pitch in, as long as the finish line was near the restaurant, at Canal Park near the Aerial Lift Bridge [which is the largest vertical lift bridge in the world and dominates the Duluth skyline].

"In 1977 the first race was held, with 150 participants. After that modest start, the number of runners kept doubling each year until it was a sizable event. [The participation of leading Minnesota distance runners Dick Beardsley and Garry Bjorklund no doubt helped burnish the run's early reputation. Today, the event's half marathon bears Bjorklund's name.] The race was sponsored by Grandma's. But in 1986, there were some high winds at the finish line, and a tent blew over. No one was hurt, but the restaurant decided it didn't want the liability for the event, so a nonprofit was created to administrate the race." Today, the event has a staff of nine, and Grandma's—which added two more Duluth locations—is still a sponsor. The North Shore Striders, which had become defunct in the 1980s, was recently revived, courtesy of seed money from Grandma's Marathon.

Unlike many marathons, Grandma's is run on a Saturday, rather than a Sunday, "so people can really celebrate once they're done, and have a day to recuperate without having to take a day off from work," Kate explained. The festivities begin on Friday with the most-of-the-day Michelina's All-You-Can-Eat Spaghetti Dinner. That evening there's a concert with a national act (in 2017, the band was Everclear) to help get runners and fans alike revved up. The race begins on Saturday in Two Harbors, to the east. Shuttle buses can

DESTINATION

37

deliver runners to the starting line; for one thousand early risers, there's the option of taking a train that follows the coastline to Two Harbors—ideal for putting you in a running state of mind. "The course makes its way along the shore of Lake Superior, through gently rolling woods," Kate said. "It starts at a slightly higher elevation than where it ends; Duluth's Aerial Lift Bridge is in your sight line much of the race. En route, runners pass over thirty-two streams that run into the lake. [Some runners will no doubt find themselves humming Gordon Lightfoot's "The Wreck of the Edmund Fitzgerald," though a happier fate awaits.] Around mile twenty, you come into the Duluth city limits. Shortly after comes Lemon Drop Hill, the biggest climb on the course. The race finishes in Canal Park after a long straightaway, near Grandma's, in the shadow of the bridge. There's a jubilant crowd waiting to greet you. Volunteers are waiting with chicken broth, fresh fruit, and other treats, and there are free massages available. Another main-stage concert follows in the evening.

"More than a few runners will opt to jump into Lake Superior after crossing the finish line. The lake, I can assure you, will be cold."

KATE KUCINSKI is the public relations and marketing director for Grandma's Marathon.

If You Go

▶ **Getting There:** Duluth is served by several carriers, including Delta (800-221-1212; delta.com) and Allegiant Air (allegiantair.com).
▶ **Best Time to Visit:** Grandma's Marathon is generally held on the third Saturday in June.
▶ **Race Information:** You'll find detailed information about the race at the Grandma's Marathon website (218-727-0947; grandmasmarathon.com).
▶ **Accommodations:** The Holiday Inn & Suites (800-477-7089; hiduluth.com) is the official lodging sponsor for the race. Other options are highlighted at Visit Duluth (800-438-5884; visitduluth.com).

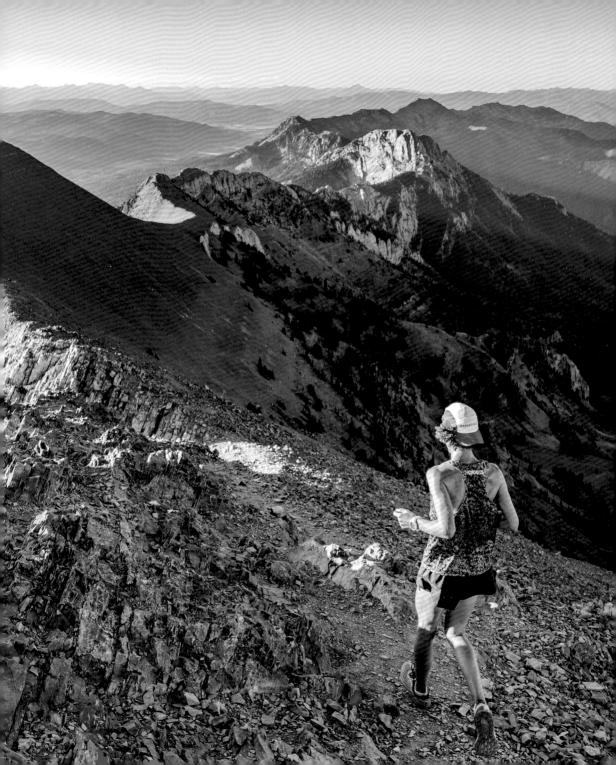

BRIDGER RIDGE RUN

RECOMMENDED BY **David Summerfield**

Broad, smooth, sheltered, and clearly marked trails. Gradual climbs and descents. Mild, consistent weather. If these qualities capture your idea of a great trail run, you'd do well to scamper in the opposite direction of the Bridger Ridge Run.

"I grew up in Switzerland, and I was drawn to the circuit of mountain races that were run in the Alps," David Summerfield began. "The Europeans are rabid about trail running and are very competitive. They don't think twice about cutting over switch-backs, and they love the steepest trails possible, dangerous stream crossings, snow-storms. It's no-holds-barred. Races were held high in the Alps, and the whole valley would turn out to watch. When I ran the old course of what would become the Ultra-Trail du Mont-Blanc, it snowed, and many runners got hypothermia. I thought my life was in danger the whole time, but it was enjoyable. Soon after I moved to Bozeman, I discovered the Bridger Ridge Run. My first year in '94, there was no real trail. You'd get up to the ridge and get to the end as best as you can. The Bridger Ridge was the first run I experienced in the States that came close to what I had experienced in Europe."

Bridger Ridge rests a few miles east of Bozeman, which is home to Montana State University (MSU) and is increasingly recognized as a four-season outdoor recreation mecca. It was an MSU Bobcat—Professor Ed Anacker, one-time head of the university's department of chemistry and biochemistry—who conceived the race. The Ed Anacker Bridger Ridge Run was first run in 1985. The race begins at the Fairy Lake Campground and ends either 19.65 or 20.55 miles later—depending on whether participants run straight down the mountain toward the finish line or take a more circuitous (and slightly safer) route. "The first few years, twenty or thirty folks would turn up," David continued. "But now the word has gotten out. We limit the race to 250 runners. I'd say that 85 per-

OPPOSITE:
At times, the trail is barely discernible along Bridger Ridge, where runners are extremely exposed to the whims of Mother Nature.

DESTINATION

38

cent of the runners are from Montana, Idaho, and Wyoming. The Big Sky Wind Drinkers [the local running club that orchestrates the event] want to maintain a local flavor.

"We have three orientation meetings the day before the race. I try my best to scare people and encourage them to be careful. Our thirty-second running was in 2016, and we had our first two helicopter evacuations, both life-threatening situations—because people did stupid things."

The course starts off with a bang as runners gain 1,800 feet on the 2.5-mile climb to Sacagawea Peak (elevation 9,604 feet), where mountain goats are likely waiting to salute your early accomplishment. "Many people get psyched when they reach Sacagawea, as you've made one-eighth of the run in less than an hour," David described. "This is one of the most scenic points of the race, as you're at the highest point. In Montana, you don't have too many mountains above timberline. On the Bridger Ridge trail, everything above eight thousand feet is above timberline. Soon after, you reach a boulder field that never seems to end. [This is the kind of shin-scraping, ankle-twisting terrain that's helped make the Bridger Ridge infamous.] Ross Peak is ahead, but it's way too technical to run. You have to drop down two thousand feet to circle around Ross and climb one thousand feet to get back to the ridge. This is mostly on talus; you'll have to watch carefully for markers, as there's no real trail. The ridges are spectacular—not exactly a knife's edge, they are a few feet across, and you wouldn't free-fall off the edge. But you're extremely exposed." Next, you'll pass over several more peaks—including Saddle, Bridger, and Baldy. After Baldy, you'll drop off the ridge toward the big white *M*. Here, you need to decide whether you'll go for the longer (but safer) trail or the steep path. A barbecue, music, and hot tubs await at the finish line.

Uneven footing, rigorous elevation gains (and drops), and a not-so-obvious trail combine to make the Bridger Ridge one of America's most technical trail runs. But the greatest provocateur on the trail may be Mother Nature, as David recounted. "We've had snowstorms during the run, fog where you couldn't see more than twenty feet, and we were losing people left and right. On one race day, I was on the ridge about thirty minutes from Baldy and could see a big black cloud coming from the west. There were little puffy clouds below the big cloud, which means either a tornado or incredible hail. I got a call from the finish line saying that they'd just heard a report from the National Weather Service calling for a life-threatening storm to hit the mountain; we had to clear off. I told them we couldn't—that runners were strung out for ten miles. I've lived through many storms, have been knocked down by lightning. You learn how not to lose your head in such situations, because you can't; the stakes are too high. I told the folks at the finish line that I had it taken care of; I knew I'd have to get off the ridge if the storm hit. It looked dire. Rain started falling, and the storm was very visible. But then it veered off to the right, just as it began to reach the range.

"An experience like that gives you a heightened sense of what the race can be about. That beating nature is more important than beating last year's time."

DAVID SUMMERFIELD is the race director of the Bridger Ridge Run and writes monthly articles for the "mature runner" in the Big Sky Wind Drinkers' newsletter. David earned his BA in philosophy and religion from Principia College, did graduate studies in French at the University of Colorado and Middlebury College, and earned a graduate degree in eighteenth-century French literature from the University of Lausanne in Switzerland. He taught French at the University of Colorado, Principia College, and Whatcom Community College. David was also the cross-country and track coach at Principia College, an NCAA Division III school. He was an instructor for the National Outdoor Leadership School's summer wilderness and winter mountaineering courses in Lander, Wyoming, and started the mountaineering program for Adventure Unlimited's youth camps in Buena Vista, Colorado. He has conducted educational and personal development tours in France, Switzerland, and the Soviet Union.

If You Go

▶ **Getting There:** Bozeman is served by a number of carriers, including Alaska Airlines (800-252-7522; alaskaair.com) and United (800-864-8331; united.com).

▶ **Best Time to Visit:** The Bridger Ridge Run is held in mid-August. The trail is generally open—and mostly clear of snow—from June through September.

▶ **Race Information:** Details about the Bridger Ridge Run reside at winddrinkers.org. The race is limited to 250 participants; interested parties must apply online.

▶ **Accommodations:** The Bozeman Convention & Visitors Bureau (406-586-5421; bozemancvb.com) lists lodging options around the Gallatin Valley.

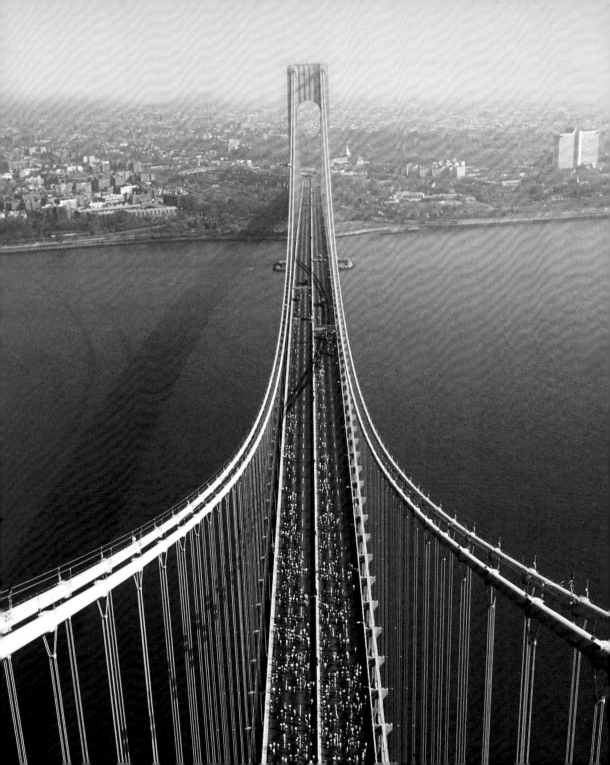

NEW YORK CITY MARATHON

RECOMMENDED BY **Peter Ciaccia**

As race director for the Tata Consultancy Services New York City Marathon, Peter Ciaccia oversees the daunting logistical challenges of coordinating the world's largest marathon in one of the world's busiest cities. A joy of the job is making a great experience for runners, spectators, and the city as a whole. "We have the ability to create something special, to continue to elevate the experience while delivering a safe and fun race," Peter began. "Everything in between is just icing on the cake. We see ourselves as producers with the goal of creating an entertainment, an event. We're always looking at the event in bits and pieces and finding ways to make incremental improvements."

The TCS New York City Marathon has certainly come a long way since 127 runners (126 men and one woman) set out to complete four loops of Central Park in 1970; fifty-five runners finished, taking home repurposed bowling and baseball trophies and cheap watches as their prizes. By 1976, Fred Lebow, who spearheaded the first race with Vince Chiappetta and the New York Road Runners (NYRR), had taken the race to the streets—literally—forging a route that encompasses all five boroughs. While the route has been modified over the years, it still takes in all five boroughs in an effort to celebrate the many faces and neighborhoods of one of the world's most diverse cities. "If you really want to get a sense of the fabric of New York, run the marathon," Peter added. "You can't help but feel the excitement of the city. It's a 26.2-mile adrenaline rush. As 39 percent of our participants are international, you get a chance to meet people from around the world. The TCS New York City Marathon is where the world comes to run."

The course of the TCS New York City Marathon begins with runners crossing from Staten Island to Brooklyn over the Verrazano Bridge. The next fourteen miles proceed north through Brooklyn and into Queens, jag west to cross into Manhattan, then continue

OPPOSITE:
Runners cross from Staten Island to Brooklyn over the Verrazano–Narrows Bridge, bringing runners to the second of five boroughs covered in the New York City Marathon.

DESTINATION

39

north into the Bronx for 1.5 miles before returning south into Manhattan, passing though Harlem and into Central Park, where the race finishes near West Sixty-Seventh Street. There are more than 135 bands on stages in all five boroughs and more than one million spectators. One of the significant changes to the race was the adoption of a wave start. "I had run the marathon before 2001 and didn't like the course that much," Peter continued. "There was a choke point at mile eight; it was so crowded, I'd have to walk. In 2001, after 9/11, there were fewer runners, and I was able to actually run through mile eight. That was when we began thinking about implementing wave starts. It took five or six years to figure this out and build the proper algorithms. We had to convince the city authorities that this would be a smarter way to proceed without impacting the reopening of the bridges and roads. They let us try it, and everyone was happy with the results."

One of the quintessential moments of the TCS New York City Marathon comes between miles fifteen and sixteen, when runners first cross into Manhattan. "When runners are coming across the Queensboro Bridge, it's a very quiet, almost introspective point of the run," Peter explained. "You know you're coming into the meat of the miles, where the race really unfolds if you're a competitor. In that silence, as you're running up the bridge, you can almost hear people next to you thinking about what's coming next. As you cross the bridge and start to descend, there's a barely audible gurgling that's starting to happen. By the time you come off the ramp onto First Avenue, the roar is deafening. Spectators are ten deep. It's easy to get excited and start running too fast up First, forgetting that you have another ten miles to go." Another favorite stretch comes around mile twenty-one, as runners come into Harlem. "From 135th to 110th [Streets], there are so many people, it feels like the Tour de France," Peter enthused.

For Peter, the most emotional part of the race arrives as he awaits the last finisher. "We have folks out on the course to keep track of where the last finisher is throughout the race," Peter said. "We'll hang around until whatever time the last finisher comes through. If the sweep buses need to come through, the remaining participants will go on the sidewalks in order to finish the race. With the help of the Department of Parks and Recreation and the NYPD, we'll keep the finish line inside Central Park open. There have been a few times when we've been there as late as midnight.

"In 2016, I had to attend the pro athlete dinner at seven; my operations team said they thought the last runner would be coming in around seven thirty. I went to the dinner, said hello to everyone, and then announced that I had to leave the dinner to wait for one of the last runners. It was a gentleman named Jonathan Mendes, ninety-six years old. He'd flown dive-bombers for the Marine Corps in World War II. It took him eleven hours and twenty minutes, but he made it across the finish line at 8:14 P.M. It was a great feeling to be able to put a medal around his neck. The professional runners didn't know about our tradition of greeting the last finishers. They were enthralled with the idea. Next year, they might come out and be part of it."

PETER CIACCIA is NYRR's president of events and the TCS New York City Marathon's race director. Under his leadership, NYRR's impact in each of the city's boroughs has deepened with the development of free community-based runs and walks and the creation of more opportunities for young runners in the calendar of NYRR races. As race director, Peter oversees the recruitment of all professional athletes in NYRR's major races and is actively directing NYRR's #RunClean, an educational initiative to address the issue of doping in the sport. Before joining NYRR, he held executive positions in the music industry for CBS Records and Sony Music Entertainment. For ten years, Peter was the owner, president, and CEO of PC Management Inc., a firm that specialized in artist development and international touring. He has been widely recognized for his efforts, including being named one of New York City's "Responsible 100" and one of *Runner's World*'s "50 Most Influential People in Running." With a lifetime passion for fitness, Peter has completed numerous marathons and ultramarathons all over the world.

If You Go

▶ **Getting There:** New York is served by most major carriers.
▶ **Best Time to Visit:** The TCS New York City Marathon is held the first Sunday in November.
▶ **Race Information:** The TCS New York City Marathon website (tcsnycmarathon.org) provides comprehensive information about the event.
▶ **Accommodations:** The New York Hilton Midtown (855-760-0871; hilton.com) and the Sheraton New York Hotel & Towers (888-627-7067; sheratonnewyork.com) serve as headquarters for race participants.

DESTINATION

39

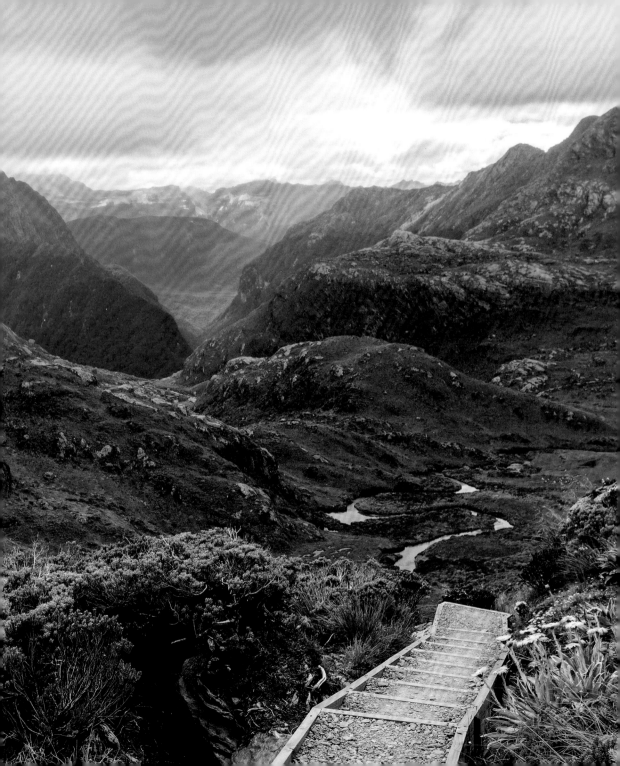

ROUTEBURN TRACK AND BEYOND

RECOMMENDED BY **Jason Schlarb**

A few years back, Jason Schlarb spent five months cycling around New Zealand's South Island. He liked it well enough to return twice more for running-oriented adventures. He's yet to be disappointed.

"If you live in the northern hemisphere and are looking for a winter mountain trail-running escape, it's hard to beat the South Island," Jason began. "There's such a diversity of running experiences available. On the west coast, there's the lush rain forest and places where glaciers come to within a few hundred yards of the ocean. Then you have volcanoes and mountains, some with glaciers. You can also run in the high desert in the eastern sections of the Otago region, where the mountains create a rain shadow. All these dramatic environments are within six to eight hours of each other. You can't get that in Colorado—or really anywhere else. Another thing that's nice about the South Island is that there aren't thousands of trail runners all over. There just aren't many people, period, so you don't have any crowds like you might find in some parts of the Dolomites or the Rockies. Because of this—and the fact that the New Zealand Department of Conservation doesn't have tremendous manpower—the trails aren't always that well maintained. Once you're off one of the Great Walks [New Zealand's premier hiking trails, or 'tramping tracks,' to borrow the Kiwi vernacular], things get a little spotty. The path is not always cut-and-dry; you need to know where you're going. The weather is also highly changeable; the wind can be quite strong. For me, the South Island has a quiet adventure feeling."

Peter Jackson's Lord of the Rings trilogy showed the world what most Kiwis already knew—that the South Island is an area of incomparable natural beauty. (Moviegoers will recognize many scenes from Middle-earth upon touching down here!) The combination

OPPOSITE:
The Routeburn Track is marked by great climbs and tremendous vistas of spectacular South Island scenery.

DESTINATION

40

179

of steep mountains, dark green forests, snowcapped peaks, foaming waterfalls, and fingers of blue fjords makes the region one of the most visually stunning temperate areas in the world. Anglers regularly make the pilgrimage to the South Island to fish its clear, uncrowded trout streams. Wineries are thriving in this former gold-mining area. And, as you may know, bungee jumping was conceived here. Five of New Zealand's nine Great Walks are on the South Island—Abel Tasman Coast, Heaphy, Milford, Routeburn, and Kepler. While the Milford Track is considered by many to be New Zealand's (if not the world's) most beautiful hike, if Jason had to choose only one track to return to, it would be the Routeburn.

The Routeburn Track winds through wild mountain country at the base of the Southern Alps, northwest of the adventure tourism mecca of Queenstown. The track connects two of the South Island's celebrated national parks—Fiordland and Mount Aspiring—through a high pass called Harris Saddle. The main trail was officially inaugurated as a tramping destination in 1968, when the construction of four huts along the route was completed, though its human history goes back almost five hundred years further. The local Máori people are believed to have traveled along the Routeburn River, between the Dart and Arahura Rivers, which were rich sources of *pounamu*—New Zealand jade. (The jade was used to make woodworking tools, weapons, and neck pendants called *hei-tiki* that are still popular in New Zealand. The World Heritage Area that encompasses much of the southern region of the South Island is known as *Te Wahipounamu*, or "the place of greenstone.") By the 1880s, the tourism value of the Routeburn region for outdoorsy people had been recognized. With the establishment of the New Zealand Department of Tourism in the early 1900s, work began in earnest to create the trails that people know today.

"The Routeburn is the most action-packed run you could find in a thirty-two-kilometer point-to-point trail," Jason enthused. "The trails are very well maintained, there are many great climbs, and the views are tremendous, as you're often up on ridges. You start along this meandering, aqua-blue river, surrounded by beech forests. As you run up toward the passes, there's tussock country, with big looming peaks and tremendous blue lakes below. As you come down the heavily forested west side of the mountains toward Milford Sound, the switchbacks are sharply slanted. On a clear day, you can see out to Milford Sound. As far as scenery and diversity of terrain are concerned, the Routeburn captures the South Island."

It should be mentioned that like the other Great Walks, the Routeburn has a wonderful hut system, which enables hikers to travel with less gear. Ultra-runners like Jason complete the trail in less than a day with no overnights necessary. "The biggest logistical challenge is arranging a car shuttle so you can get back to Queenstown," he added. "And beware of the sand fleas at the pickup zone. You don't want to have to wait there long!"

A very different, yet hardly less appealing run awaits you near the top of the South Island at Abel Tasman National Park, which extends from Wainui Inlet in the north to Marahau in the south and includes the waters of the Tonga Island Marine Reserve. Two well-known tracks traverse the park, including the aforementioned sixty-kilometer Tasman Coast Track. "Abel Tasman doesn't have the dramatic glaciers and mountain passes that you find in the south, but it has beautiful empty golden-sand beaches and a nicely maintained single track overlooking headlands and the ocean. It's a bit more crowded than Routeburn [Abel Tasman is New Zealand's busiest national park], but people are very friendly. At one point, there's a tidal crossing, and you need to consult tide tables to time it correctly; I was strongly advised against trying to swim across. I think this is a cool aspect of the walk. At the end of the run, there are boats for hire to take you back to the starting point. There are colonies of fur seals in the north." If you're moving a bit slower, there are four huts and many campgrounds along the Tasman Coast Track; Jason completed his run of Abel Tasman in a day.

"A great element of running on the South Island is the kindness of the people," Jason shared. "They are very modest, open, and trustworthy. I met one woman when I was getting ready to do a run and mentioned that I would be doing the Kepler Track in a few weeks. Without hesitation, she offered me the use of a family cabin near the track's beginning. That sort of generosity typifies the South Island spirit."

JASON SCHLARB is a professional mountain, trail, and ultra-runner who lives in a cabin near Durango, Colorado. In 2016, Jason was cochampion with Kilian Jornet at the Hardrock 100, which he has won twice, and he holds the course record at the Run Rabbit Run 100 in Colorado; he was fourth (and the first American finisher) in the 2014 UTMB, and has accumulated many other national and international running accomplishments and accolades. His sponsors include Altra Footwear, Smartwool, Vitargo, Flora, Ultimate Direction, Julbo Eyewear, and EPIC Bar. Jason served ten years active duty in the US Air

Force before separating as a major. Jason is also a performance coach; learn more about him and his services at jasonschlarb.com, and follow Jason on Instagram: @jasonschlarb.

▶ **Getting There:** Visitors fly into Queenstown, which is served by Air New Zealand (800-262-1234; airnewzealand.com) and Jetstar (866-397-8170; jetstar.com) via Auckland and Christchurch.

▶ **Best Time to Visit:** December, January, and February comprise the austral summer and are fine times to visit, though fairly clement conditions prevail from October to April.

▶ **Running Information:** The New Zealand Department of Conservation (+64 32498514; doc.govt.nz) highlights many of the trails on the South Island, including the Routeburn Track. Jason also recommends some of the fine trails right outside Queenstown, and the Motatapu Ultra Run—a "beastly point-to-point 50K, one of a kind!"

▶ **Accommodations:** Destination Queenstown (+64 34410700; queenstown-nz.co.nz) lists accommodations in the region's hub town. New Zealand Tourism (newzealand.com) highlights options around the South Island.

DESTINATION

40

EUGENE HASH

RECOMMENDED BY **Christina Howard**

Eugene, Oregon, is a hallowed place in American running circles. It was in this southern Willamette Valley town that Bill Bowerman coached the University of Oregon Ducks to four NCAA titles and, with the help of a former miler named Phil Knight, started a little shoe company that would come to be called Nike. It was also here, under Bowerman's guidance, that Steve "Pre" Prefontaine came to prominence. Hayward Field, home of the U of O's track and field teams, is the frequent host of USA Track & Field championships, NCAA championships, and Olympic Trials, as well as the annual Nike Prefontaine Classic.

Each Sunday afternoon, Eugene is also home to a slightly different style of event—the Eugene Hash.

Christina Howard was introduced to the Hash House Harriers after finishing graduate school in San Francisco. "A friend wanted to do a hash in Marin County and didn't want to go alone," she explained. "I was happy to go along. She canceled at the last minute, but I went anyway, though I didn't know any of the people. It was like a scavenger hunt with running and beer. The other participants were fun and silly, and running on trails, I got to see parts of Marin I'd never seen. Though all the runners were fifteen years older, they welcomed me like an old friend. I began going most Mondays. Eventually I got my hash name—Headqueen. (Most hashes have a naming tradition; at the time I was working with patients with brain trauma, hence mine.) I also met my husband.

"Hashers from all over would come to San Francisco for the Bay to Breakers. It was a big bacchanalia. We met some hashers from Eugene and became friends. When my husband and I moved up, the Eugene hashers were my instant friends. I bought some rain gear, as Oregon would be a little wetter than the Bay Area, and began hashing on Sundays."

DESTINATION

41

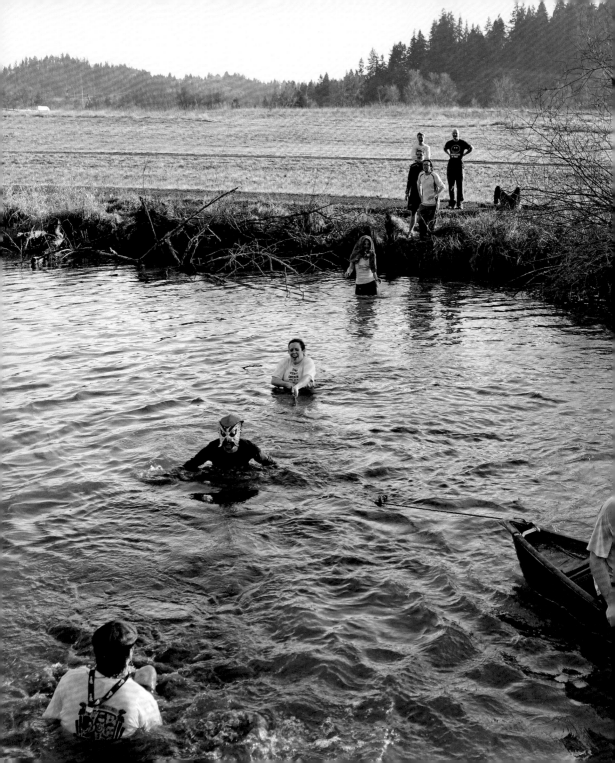

The idea of hashing has its roots in an old English schoolboy game called Hare and Hounds. As told by the Sarnia chapter of the Hash House Harriers:

OPPOSITE:
Eugene hashes
are often
determined on
the fly and may
not adhere to
traditional paths.

> Some players, called "hounds," chase others, called "hares," who have left a trail of paper scraps along their route across fields, hedges, streams, bogs, and hills. Hare and Hounds as an adult sport began in the fall of 1867 with a group of London oarsmen who wanted to keep fit during the winter. Also called "Paper Chasing" or the "Paper Chase," the game became very popular after its introduction on Wimbledon Common in 1868 by the Thames Hare and Hounds. Early clubs called themselves "Hare and Hounds" or simply "Harriers."

Modern hashing can be traced to Kuala Lumpur in 1937, where an English transplant named Albert Stephen Ignatius Gispert assembled several other expatriates for a harrier group. Hash House—the nickname for the Selangor Club, where many of the men lived—became the group's moniker. The group's 1938 charter set out its philosophy:

1. To promote physical fitness among our members
2. To get rid of weekend hangovers
3. To acquire a good thirst and to satisfy it in beer
4. To persuade the older members that they are not as old as they feel

The magic combination of running, a boys' game, and beer had obvious appeal, and the idea of hashing slowly spread. It's estimated there are nearly two thousand hashes in 180 countries . . . including the Eugene Hash.

"The Eugene run is held on Sundays," Christina continued, "and on a given day usually has twenty to twenty-five people. Each hash has its own culture. Some are more running-centered than party-centered; that's the case in Eugene. Hashers from other places and newcomers are welcome to join. If it's a 'live trail,' the hare is given a fifteen-minute head start to mark the trail with flour or chalk. Before the hare leaves, though, there are introductions and a blessing from the hash's religious adviser. Then the hashers take off, trying to find the trail. Eugene has a great urban trail system and many small parks. You can expect to run on dirt for a good portion of the hash. At this point, everyone is calling, 'Are you?' as in, 'Are you on the trail?' When someone finds the first mark, they'll call, 'On one'; when they find a second, 'On two'; when they find a third, it's 'On on,' and you know someone's on the real trail. Sometimes the hare will leave false trails—the mark for this is three thick lines, which means YBF (you've been . . . fooled). Then you have to go back. Halfway through the game, which usually spans four and a half to six miles, there's a beer check. This is indicated by the letters BN (beer near) on the ground. That means there's a twelve-pack or two under a bush nearby. There is decorum at a beer check—you don't leave until everyone has a beer. You don't drink and run.

"Hashes are A to B runs in Eugene. At the end, someone will generally have a simple meal prepared—chili, a sandwich bar, make your own burrito. There will be more beer. Then there will generally be a 'down-down' or two. This is when someone is punished for a 'crime' perpetrated on the trail, like talking too much about work or wearing a shirt from a running event. You have to either drink a beer or wear it."

The Eugene hashers have several signature events. One involves dressing as clowns. Another is timed to coincide with the Prefontaine Classic. "We all wear press-on moustaches and vintage track shirts," Christina said. "We make sure to stop at Pre's Rock, a shrine of sorts where many runners leave mementos. It's a beer stop."

CHRISTINA HOWARD is a cofounder of Axis Physical Therapy and Rehab in Eugene. She holds a master's degree in physical therapy from the University of San Francisco and San Francisco State University and estimates that she has participated in five hundred hashes since her first in 1995.

If You Go

▶ **Getting There:** Eugene is served by a number of carriers, including Alaska Airlines (800-252-7522; alaskaair.com) and United (800-864-8331; united.com).

▶ **Best Time to Visit:** Hashes are held year-round. Visits from late spring to mid-fall are less likely to encounter rain. The Prefontaine Memorial Hash is held in late May.

▶ **More Information:** Visit facebook.com/groups/EugeneH3 to learn about upcoming hashes in the Eugene area.

▶ **Accommodations:** Travel Lane County (800-547-5445; eugenecascadescoast.org) lists lodging options around Eugene.

HOOD TO COAST

RECOMMENDED BY **Felicia Hubber**

"My father, Bob Foote, loves to run, loves to ski, and enjoys spending time on the Oregon coast," Felicia Hubber recalled. "Back in 1982, he wanted to figure out a way to combine these activities while creating an opportunity to have a fun running weekend with his friends. He came up with the idea of the Hood to Coast relay and pitched it to the Oregon Road Runners Club. They agreed to produce the first event. That first year, there were eight teams with ten runners each. My dad was an architect and a bit of a perfectionist. He wheel-measured every five-mile increment to determine exactly where the exchange of batons had to occur—even if it was the middle of a busy intersection. At the time, he thought they'd be lucky if it happened a second year. He spent so many all-nighters trying to bring the event off that he felt terrible during the actual running. But everyone had a blast. The race created a sense of camaraderie, friendship, and inspiration beyond expectations. It grew from eight teams in year one, to sixty-four the following year, subsequently 150, 237, 408, and then 500 teams. It was capped at five hundred for a while, but there were so many requests, the capacity was expanded to a limit of 1,050 teams. All this was through word of mouth. A participant might step into a van not knowing everyone on the team; twenty-four hours later, you might have a new best friend or a life partner. Today, the Hood to Coast is the largest relay race in the world."

The Hood to Coast, held in late August each year, traverses 199 miles. It begins at the highest paved point of the Beaver State's tallest mountain—Timberline Lodge (6,000 feet) on Mount Hood (11,234 feet)—and continues west, descending through the foothills of the Cascades, crossing the fertile Willamette Valley (including the city of Portland), climbing up and down Oregon's Coast Range, before reaching the Pacific at the town of Seaside . . . and one of the West Coast's biggest beach parties. Teams of eight to twelve runners (twelve is

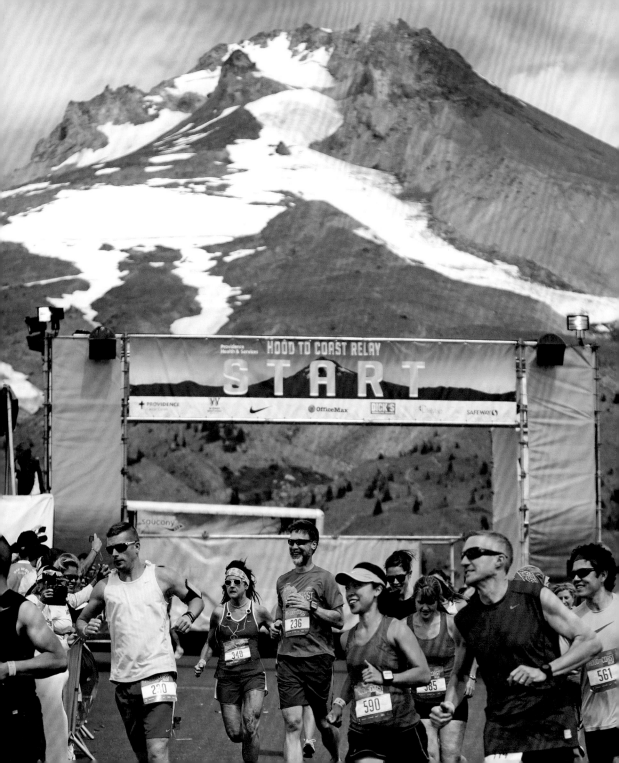

most common) divide up thirty-six legs; legs vary from 3.48 to 7.72 miles, and each team member must complete at least three legs. "We get a broad range of runners participating in the Hood to Coast," Felicia continued. "Some are elite runners; others are weekend joggers who are undertaking the biggest running challenge in their life. While we get a lot of complete teams registering, there are often teams that have places for people who want to run but don't have a team. [Social media has greatly simplified filling out teams!] Teams can break up the legs as they wish; generally, more seasoned runners are given the more difficult stretches. As one runner is covering his or her leg, the team van goes ahead to the next exchange point. Vans are stocked with snacks and beverages, and teams will listen to music and share stories along the way. Depending on timing, some teams will even stop and have dinner in a restaurant while a leg is being run."

OPPOSITE: The Hood to Coast is the world's largest relay race, covering 199 miles from Timberline Lodge on Mount Hood (shown here) to Seaside.

On the Friday that the relay begins, the first wave of runners takes off from Timberline Lodge on Mount Hood at five A.M. (Timberline Lodge, a marvel of Depression-era Civilian Conservation Corps design and construction, might look familiar in the early dawn light; its exterior was used in the Stanley Kubrick thriller *The Shining*.) Felicia described the events that follow. "Emmy Award–winning reporter John Hammarley is our announcer. He gets the teams amped up as they shoot down the mountain. Runners on that first leg lose two thousand feet in the first 5.5 miles. It can be brutal if you don't know how to tackle such a downhill. If you run it lighter, you don't even feel like you're running. The first four legs of the race are all downhill, through the Mount Hood National Forest. As the sun's coming up, there's snow-topped Mount Hood lit up behind you. Around leg six, you come into the town of Sandy, and then you pop out into farmland, rolling terrain with pasture land, and tree farms. By leg eight and the town of Boring, you come to the Springwater Corridor, a former rail line that has been converted to a multiuse trail and leads right into Portland. You cross the Willamette River on the Hawthorne Bridge [one of twelve bridges that cross the river] and then head through an industrial area. As you head west, you'll pass through a series of small river communities that flank the Columbia River—Linnton, Scappoose, St. Helens [which looks across the Columbia to the volcano of the same name that erupted in 1980]. Many schools in these towns hold fund-raisers at this time, offering food, showers, or sleeping accommodations, and they are patronized by our participants.

"Once you've gotten past St. Helens, you come into a thickly forested area of the course as you head into the Coast Range. Night has fallen, and some stretches of the road

DESTINATION

42

FIFTY PLACES TO RUN BEFORE YOU DIE

here are gravel. There are no neighborhoods, no streetlights. It can be pitch-black, though we require participants to have reflective vests and front and back flashlights. For team members who are running this leg, it can be a very Zen experience. You almost feel like you're running in a black hole. The fastest teams are coming out of the Coast Range just as the sun is rising. Runners descend into the town of Seaside, run twelve blocks on the Seaside Promenade parallel to the Pacific, then cut down to the finish line on the beach. The first finishers come in around seven A.M.; the last team is generally in by eight P.M. There's a massive beach party at the run's conclusion—sixty thousand to seventy thousand people—with local beer, wines, and live music. Even though people have been up for thirty-six hours, they're dancing, running on endorphins."

Felicia has attended more than thirty Hood to Coasts, notching her first when she was three months old. One of her most powerful memories is of the first time her husband ran the event with her. "My husband is a non-runner, but he wanted to experience the event before he came to work for the race," she said. "We assembled a group of friends; he ran the shortest legs, and he was handing off to me for each of our three rotations. My husband has MS, so it was very important for him to do this. He completed them all and was on his last leg—leg thirty-two—which comes just after you come out of the Coast Range. He was coming up a hill to exchange and hand off to me, limping with tiredness as he approached the handoff. It was a breathtaking moment, as I could see the mix of agony and pride on his face in having accomplished such a monumental endeavor. I think that's how many people feel in taking on the Hood to Coast."

FELICIA HUBBER has been president of the Hood to Coast organization since 2006. An avid runner, she has participated in the race six times and has attended or assisted in the race for thirty-two of the thirty-five years it has been in existence. The first leg of the race is Felicia's favorite, and she climbed to the peak of Mount Hood a month before the Hood to Coast for inspiration. Felicia began running at age nine and has calculated that her lifetime mileage is equivalent to nearly one and a half times the circumference of the earth. She treks abroad regularly and makes a point to eat Indian food and run in every country she visits.

DESTINATION

42

If You Go

► **Getting There:** Portland is served by most major carriers. Alaska Airlines (800-252-7522; alaskaair.com) offers discounted air travel for the event.

► **Best Time to Visit:** The Hood to Coast is generally held the last weekend in August. Portland has clement weather most of the year, though November through April is often wet.

► **Race Information:** The Hood to Coast usually fills up the day registration opens, though spots are almost always available for runners without a team. Visit hoodtocoastrelay.com for details.

► **Accommodations:** Travel Portland (travelportland.com) lists lodging options around the Rose City for the race's start. The City of Seaside Visitors Bureau (seasideor.com) details lodging near the finish. Travel Oregon (traveloregon.com) is a clearinghouse for lodging throughout the state.

DESTINATION

42

191

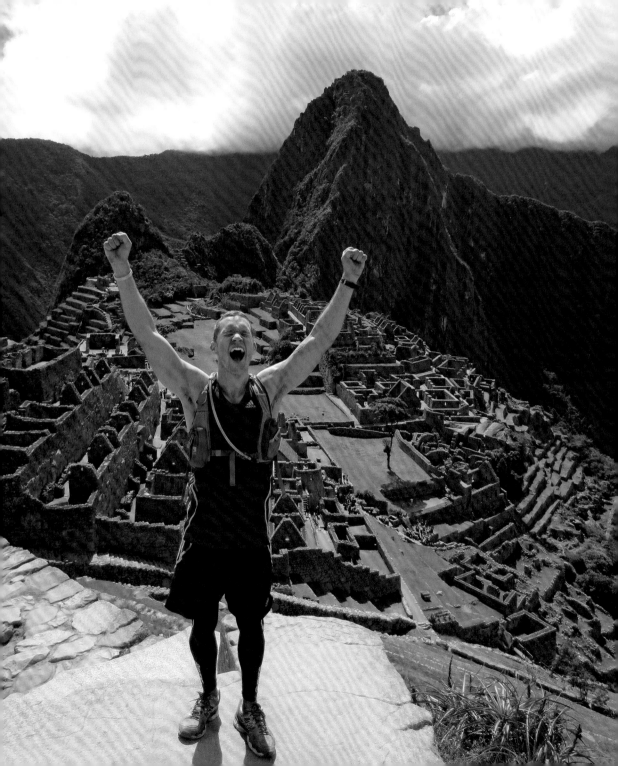

INCA TRAIL

RECOMMENDED BY **Bill Hoffman**

Had you told Bill Hoffman a decade ago that he'd one day be running through the Andes to Machu Picchu, he likely would've laughed. "I have flat feet and bad Achilles tendons and had never been a runner at all," Bill recalled. "Then I read *Born to Run*. At the time, I was an overweight, middle-aged guy at a desk. After reading the book, I bought a pair of those toe shoes and ran a mile. My knees didn't hurt. I'd run a mile a day in the woods behind my house, then two, then three, then five. Next I did a few ten-mile runs, and a friend suggested that it was marathon time. I was eleven months into my running career, and I did it—four hours and thirty-six minutes. I learned from the experience, and six months later, I ran an hour faster and soon after qualified for the Boston Marathon. Training for Boston, a friend told me about an ultramarathon in the Adirondacks. That got me into trail running . . . and that's what brought me to the Inca Trail."

The trek along the Inca Trail to Machu Picchu sits high in the pantheon of bucket-list adventures for many ardent hikers. It traces a section of the path of an old Inca roadway that led from Cusco to Machu Picchu, in the Andes of southern Peru. The Inca Trail—as utilized by modern-day trekkers—begins at the town of Piskacucho and stretches some twenty-nine miles. The scenery is breathtaking; high above the rushing Urubamba and Cusichaka Rivers, the trail passes through a variety of habitats—from alpine forest to cloud forest (rain forest with a perpetual cover of clouds at the canopy level) to pampas above the tree line—and traces the edge of the Vilcabamba mountain range, whose highest peak, Salcantay, looms overhead at 20,574 feet.

Since 1996, runners have been able to compete in an informal (though supported) marathon, covering much of the trail in one fell swoop. Along the way, there's a chance to gain a greater understanding of Incan culture as well as your boundaries as a runner.

OPPOSITE:
The Inca Trail takes runners as high as 13,779 feet. Finishers have reason to celebrate!

DESTINATION

43

After landing in Lima, runners gather for a flight to Cusco, the site of many architectural wonders from the Inca Empire. Cusco rests at 11,150 feet; a few days here allow you to acclimatize to the altitude, one of many challenges posed by the Inca Marathon. "I had arrived a day earlier than the other runners," Bill continued, "and though there wasn't a run scheduled, I talked my way into doing a run with the guides. The next day, we had a tour of some of Cusco's sites and another run. There were participants from all over the world—including New Zealand, Japan, and Spain. Having the opportunity to get your legs moving at that altitude and to get to know the guides, porters, and other runners made the experience feel safe and comfortable." From Cusco, the runners travel to Urubamba in the Sacred Valley of the Incas. After more sight-seeing and a few more acclimatization runs on area trails, participants move on to the Inca Trail and prepare for the marathon or 30K.

The day before the marathon, participants (and accompanying friends and family members) are brought to the Inca Trail at kilometer eighty-two. From here, it's roughly a five-mile hike (or run) to the camp at Llactapata, elevation 8,400 feet. "There were sixty or seventy porters involved, and when we arrived, tents were all set up," Bill recalled. "We had a nice lunch and dinner and tried to get to bed early. We were awoken at two A.M., had breakfast, and then hiked up to the starting point with head lamps. The race began at four A.M. The first climb was on a smooth single track, and I made ten or twelve miles in two hours. I remember looking at the time, thinking that we were on track to be breaking some records . . . but not realizing that the toughest part of the trail—much steeper and rockier—was still ahead. When we started out, it was cloudy, but as we went along the trail the clouds cleared out and the stars appeared, illuminating the giant peaks around us. It was ominous and beautiful at the same time."

One of the most daunting points of the run comes at Warmiwañusq'a, "Dead Woman's Pass," which sits at 13,779 feet. "At that point, I wasn't running," Bill noted. "It was pretty painful. On another climb, the altitude got to me and I had to walk. I looked at my altimeter and it showed 12,500 feet. When I dropped a thousand feet, I felt better . . . though making your way down isn't always easy, as there's some rock-hopping involved. I kept thinking there would be someone coming behind me, but the next runner was an hour behind." In addition to vistas of the glaciated peaks of the Vilcabamba mountain range above and the deep gorges of the Urubamba River below, runners are treated to glimpses of Incan ruins, including the Runkurakay watchtower, the fortress of Sayacmarca, and the deserted village of Sayacmarca. Eventually, a dirt trail leads to Intipunku, "Gateway of the Sun," at 8,860 feet . . . which signals that the run is nearly done.

"As you drop down, you see the ruins of Machu Picchu and other people, and it seems like you're actually going to finish the run," Bill recalled. "The finish line is right at the spot where you can see the terraced city and Wayna Picchu rising in the background. It's a pretty amazing place to finish a race. My time was eight hours and thirty-nine minutes. I've run some fifty-mile races, and I'd say this is comparable.

"My family hiked into Machu Picchu from seven miles down the trail. I beat them to the finish line, although they were able to sleep in. The next day, after a tour of Machu Picchu, we hiked to the top of Wayna Picchu."

BILL HOFFMAN is a founder of Kitware and currently serves as chairman of the board and chief technical officer. He is the original author and lead architect of CMake, an open-source, cross-platform build and configuration tool that is used by thousands of projects around the world, and he is the coauthor of the accompanying text, *Mastering CMake*. Bill received a BS in computer science from the University of Central Florida and an MS in computer science from Rensselaer Polytechnic Institute (RPI). He has planned and taught several graduate-level courses at RPI as well as a course in object-oriented programming at New York University. Bill has completed more than twenty-seven marathons and longer races, including four Boston Marathons, two JFK 50 Miles, and four Wakely Dam Ultras.

If You Go

▶ **Getting There:** Cusco is the staging area for hiking the Inca Trail; Cusco is served from Lima by several airlines, including LATAM Airlines (866-435-9526; latam.com).
▶ **Best Time to Visit:** Andes Adventures (310-395-5265; andesadventures.com) conducts unofficial Inca Trail marathons in the austral winter—June, July, and August.
▶ **Race Information:** Andes Adventures organizes a number of runs each season. They coordinate all aspects of the adventure, from lodging to guides and porters to support during the run. Each running tour is limited to forty participants.

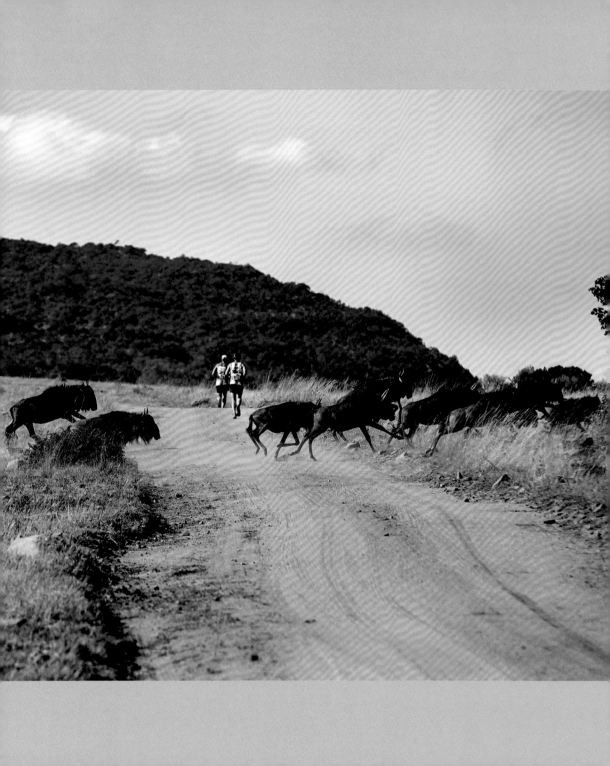

BIG FIVE MARATHON

RECOMMENDED BY **Rune Nortoft**

The chance to take part in an African game drive tends to be high on the bucket list for nature lovers and urbanites alike. On such safaris, you have the chance to encounter the Big Five—lion, elephant, Cape buffalo, leopard, and rhinoceros—with no fences or other obstructions between you and the animals. (The term "Big Five," incidentally, was first coined by hunters, who considered these five animals the most difficult to hunt on foot, and the most dangerous.) If you think that sounds thrilling, now imagine running a marathon across the terrain these noble creatures call home. If you find yourself doubly enthused, then there's a good chance the Big Five Marathon in South Africa is the trail-running adventure you've been looking for.

OPPOSITE: One will very likely encounter some four-legged runners during the Big Five Marathon—in this case, wildebeest.

"In the early 2000s, Albatros Travel was sending a lot of guests to the Limpopo region of South Africa on safaris," Rune Nortoft recalled. "We were working with someone from the Danish Athletics Federation on the Great Wall Marathon in China, and he suggested that we stage a run in a game park. Our director was dismissive, thinking it would be too difficult from a logistics perspective. But then he thought more about it and decided, 'Why not?' One of the biggest challenges would be guaranteeing the safety of our participants. We eventually found a great partner in Entabeni Safari Conservancy. The first Big Five Marathon was held in 2005."

Situated in the Limpopo province of northeastern South Africa, and more specifically in the Waterberg region (named for its many lakes, swamps, and rivers, which appear throughout an expanse that is otherwise a typical dry savanna), Entabeni Safari Conservancy is the largest of several nature preserves in Limpopo. Home, as promised, to the Big Five game animals, the conservancy's land is also interspersed with sandstone monoliths, ravines, and waterfalls, some of which come into play as you run the course.

DESTINATION

44

197

"The day before and after the run, guests have an opportunity to participate in safari drives," Rune continued. "You have a very good chance to come upon lion, elephant, buffalo, leopard, and rhino as well as giraffe and antelope on the drive. The day after your first game drive, you find yourself running through the same area. We work very hard with Entabeni's rangers to give runners the feeling that they're in a wild place, but that it's safe. There are roughly thirty rangers guarding the course. Some conduct a watch of the lion prides the night before to track their locations, and groups of rangers are assigned to follow them. They report locations in the morning so we can start the race. If the lions do start moving close to the course, we're alerted, and we'll stop the race. In 2016, we had to change the course because a lion had made a kill on the route the day before the race, and the cats won't move from a kill for four or five days. In 2015, we had to delay the start of the race for thirty minutes, as rangers had lost track of a group of lions. Their tracks suggested they were safely distant, but the rangers need to see the animals themselves to be sure."

While lions have so far failed to undermine a race in progress, pachyderms once posed a problem. "At some of the aid stations, we had bananas for runners. Some elephants were drawn to that station, and we had to close that part of the course. We had to find an extra five miles while the race was on, but we managed. We have a plan B, C, and D in place for such occasions!"

A once-over of the Big Five course that runners receive on Friday while on the game drive may leave some wondering if lions and elephants are the least of their problems. "The course is scenic but brutal," Rune described. "In some cases, you're running on game trails. In places, there's deep sand, which is very difficult to navigate. Other sections have stones of different sizes, so you need to step carefully. If you're generally a four-hour marathoner, you'll find this a five-hour course. Start time is a little later—at nine A.M.—as it's easier for rangers to locate animals. The temperatures are very comfortable for running, with a high in the sixties. The sun is always shining. We have aid stations every four kilometers with both Coca-Cola and water available. (It's common to have Coke at races in South Africa.)"

The Yellowwood Valley section of the race poses the greatest challenge. First, runners must pound down a long (two-mile), quad-killing descent; fortunately, this is on a paved surface. However, the descent is followed by a five-mile loop through deep sand . . . which brings you back to the paved surface and the climb out. "When we do the drive-through on Friday, people are shocked at the steepness of the hill. They think it will be impossible to drive it; then they realize they'll have to run it." (There's no shame in walking this section, and many participants do.) The course then enters Long Drive, a narrow valley that's mostly flat and has good, packed trails. The last few miles have some ups and downs on rocky trails before bringing you to the finish at Lakeside Lodge.

While runners will *not* see lions during the Big Five Marathon, you're fairly certain to see giraffes and rhinos in the distance, as well as antelopes.

"There aren't too many spectators at the finish line, though runners finishing earlier do hang out," Rune added. "But you don't come to run at Entabeni to have a spectator atmosphere. You're running against nature. At times, you feel like it's just you and the planet."

RUNE NORTOFT is the race director at Albatros Travel, an adventure-oriented travel company based in Denmark. In addition to Arctic cruises and safari experiences, Albatros organizes renowned marathon events such as the Great Wall Marathon, Petra Desert Marathon, Polar Circle Marathon, and Bagan Temple Marathon.

If You Go

▶ **Getting There:** Participants fly into Johannesburg, which is served by most major international carriers. Albatros Adventure Marathons coordinates transport to your lodge in Entabeni.

▶ **Best Time to Visit:** The Big Five Marathon is generally held in late June.

▶ **Race Information:** You'll find all relevant information on the Big Five at big-five-marathon.com. The limited spots for the Big Five sell out early.

▶ **Accommodations:** When you travel with Albatros (as most do), all lodging is arranged at such venues as Ravineside Lodge, Wildside Tented Camp, and Albatros Ranger Camp.

DESTINATION

44

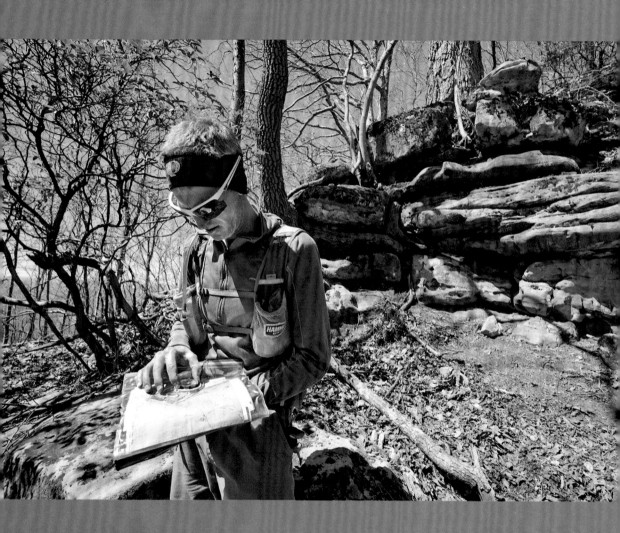

BARKLEY MARATHONS

RECOMMENDED BY **"Frozen Ed" Furtaw**

The Barkley Marathons is not quite like any other running event. For starters, the only way you can submit an entry is by hunting down someone who has competed in the Barkley in the past to acquire the race director's email address and the date on which entries must be submitted. Should you be among the lucky few whose entries are accepted (generally forty a year)—and if you're a first-timer—your application must include $1.60, a license plate from your home state, and an essay on "why I should be allowed to run the Barkley." On race day, you must be prepared to start at any time between midnight and noon; the blowing of a conch shell announces that the race will start in an hour. The official start of the race is signaled by the lighting of a cigarette.

And then there's the race itself: one hundred miles (or more) up and down several mountains in Frozen Head State Park and Natural Area, sometimes on trails, often not . . . a course so rigorous that many years no one finishes at all in the allotted sixty hours. (In thirty-one years of the Barkley Marathons, there have been only seventeen finishers; a runner named Jared Campbell has finished the race three times.)

"I first read of the Barkley Marathons in the running calendar of *UltraRunning* magazine in 1985," "Frozen Ed" Furtaw recalled. "It was advertised as a fifty-mile race with 24,850 feet of climb. I was familiar with eastern Tennessee, and I thought it was a misprint, that there couldn't be that much elevation gain. The first Barkley was held in 1986. I heard that no one finished and thought maybe it wasn't a misprint after all. I bumped into Gary Cantrell [the founder and race director for the Barkley Marathons] at another race in 1987 in Birmingham, Alabama. He showed me a topo [topographical] map of Frozen Head State Park, and there were elevation lines every sixteenth of an inch, which suggested very steep terrain. No one finished again in 1987. I was doing fifty-mile races

OPPOSITE:
The Barkley
Marathons
has more than
its share of
eccentricities,
including no
markers on the
trail . . . hence
this participant
consulting a map.

DESTINATION

45

in less than eight hours and figured that someone should be able to do the Barkley in less than twenty-four hours. I decided that I'd attempt the Barkley in 1988."

Frozen Head State Park rests in eastern Tennessee's Crab Orchard Mountains, which make up the southern edge of the Cumberland Mountains. The park (and adjacent natural area) takes in nearly twenty-five thousand acres and includes some eighty miles of trails. Frozen Head Mountain, at an elevation of 3,324 feet, looms high above the surrounding forest. (During late fall and winter, the mountain's summit is often crowned in frost or snow . . . hence its name, and Ed's nickname.) The infamous Brushy Mountain State Penitentiary once operated adjacent to Frozen Head (it was closed in 2009), and the prison played a key role in the Barkley's genesis. James Earl Ray, who murdered Martin Luther King Jr., was one of Brushy Mountain's most notorious inmates. "In 1977, Ray escaped the prison," Ed continued. "He was recaptured about fifty-four hours later and had only made it about eight miles from Brushy Mountain. The story goes that upon hearing about the escape, Gary said to his friend Karl 'Raw Dog' Henn, 'In fifty-four hours, I probably could've run a hundred miles.' Hence the idea of a hundred-mile race."

In the first few years of its existence, the Barkley Marathons (which was named in honor of Barry Barkley, a farmer and old friend of Gary's who often supported him in his ultra efforts) consisted of three loops of a course that is *roughly* twenty miles long, following the perimeter of the park; "roughly," as many participants insist it is longer. (The number of loops was increased to six in 1989, making the Barkley one hundred miles or more; these days, it's five loops.) The course changes every year, especially after a year in which there's been a successful finisher. In his fine history of the event, *Tales from Out There*, Ed describes Gary's design intent as keeping the event "at the outer limit of human possibility." In some places, the course is on hiking trails, but in many others, it's decidedly off-piste, even heading through patches of briars. There are no markers; participants get to view the course on a master map the day before the race and must make their own notes. There are also no aid stations beyond the check-ins at the end of each loop. To show that they have completed the loop to the route's specifications, participants must find books along the course and tear out (and present) the pages corresponding to their race numbers; each participant receives a new race number after each loop. Should a runner throw in the towel at some point in the race, "Taps" is played on a bugle at the end point.

What is the greatest challenge posed by the Barkley? The punishing distance? The course that meanders through the woods, often in the dark, without markers? Finding the email address of the race director? All of the above? Most of the chosen few who have participated would cite elevation as one of the more brutal elements of the race. "In 2016, the twenty-mile loop had thirteen thousand feet of climb," Ed observed. "I read a study of energy expenditure. It said that five hundred feet of elevation gain is the equivalent expenditure of one flat mile. So when you look at thirteen thousand feet, it's like adding another twenty-six miles . . . so one loop is the energy equivalent of a fifty-mile race. Though, as Gary always claims, there's no net elevation gain.

"With the Barkley, you have to redefine success. It's about the attempt rather than a finish. It's a reminder to set a goal, even if you can't ultimately reach it."

"FROZEN ED" FURTAW has been running marathons and longer races since 1978 and has completed more than one hundred ultramarathons. He was one of the most successful competitors in the early years of the Barkley Marathons. This earned him the nickname "Frozen Ed," after the Frozen Head Mountain area in Tennessee, where the Barkley Marathons is held. Now a retired engineer living in northern Arizona, Ed is the author of *Tales from Out There: The Barkley Marathons, the World's Toughest Trail Race.*

If You Go

▶ **Getting There:** The nearest major airport to Frozen Head State Park is in Knoxville (fifty miles distant), which is served by several carriers, including Delta (800-221-1212; delta.com) and United (800-864-8331; united.com).

▶ **Best Time to Visit:** The Barkley Marathons is usually held between mid-March and mid-April . . . and is dependent on the inspiration of race director Gary Cantrell.

▶ **Race Information:** As ultra-runner Matt Mahoney has noted (at mattmahoney.net/barkley), interested applicants must email the race director on a certain day of the year. (Only people who have raced it before know the email address and the day.) Good luck!

▶ **Accommodations:** Camping is available at Frozen Head State Park (tnstateparks.com). The Scenic River Inn Motel (423-346-5733) is the nearest indoor lodging.

DESTINATION

45

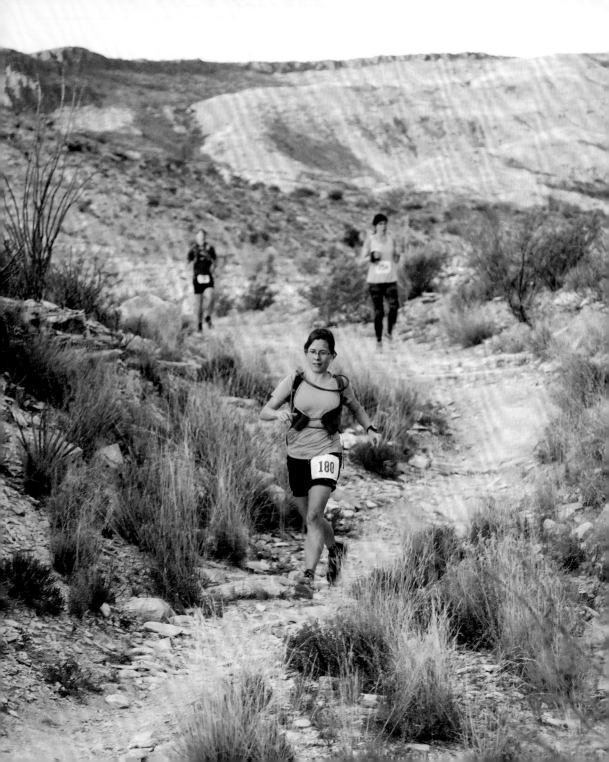

BIG BEND ULTRA

RECOMMENDED BY **P. Carroll Voss** AND **Jamie Stone**

"Everything's bigger in Texas," as the old saw goes, and this aphorism certainly speaks to the grand open spaces of Big Bend Ranch State Park. Big Bend rests in an incredibly remote part of very remote country, some 250 miles from the nearest commercial airport. The park encompasses more than three hundred thousand acres of rugged high desert along the Rio Grande (which separates the park from Mexico) in the far southwest of the Lone Star State, with rugged mountains and steep canyons dotted with creosote bush, honey mesquite, tamarisk, and many varieties of cactus; some of the early scenes in the Coen brothers' film *No Country for Old Men* give a great sense of the region's landscape. Big Bend takes its name from the point where the river turns to the northeast before assuming its long southeastern course to the Gulf of Mexico. (Together with the adjacent Big Bend National Park, Big Bend Ranch State Park is part of the largest protected swath of the Chihuahuan Desert in the United States, totaling more than one million acres. The desert extends into the Mexican states of Chihuahua, Coahuila, Durango, Zacatecas, and Nuevo Leon; from Big Bend, it stretches west across New Mexico into southeastern Arizona.) Though seemingly hostile to life, Big Bend is home to a host of animals, including javelinas (which resemble smallish wild boars but are a quite distinct species), coyotes, black bears, bighorn sheep, mountain lions, and many resident and migratory birds. Low humidity and the lack of urban light pollution make Big Bend ideal for stargazing.

It's ideal for running too, as P. Carroll Voss and Jamie Stone have learned. "The Big Bend area was discovered by trail runners from South Texas looking for single-track courses in dry, cool, and remote locations," Carroll shared. "Single-track paths traverse limestone cliffs, springs, wide and narrow creek bottoms. Fall, winter, and early spring

OPPOSITE:
The Big Bend Ultra showcases the rugged beauty of Big Bend State Park, which is also the site of the Trans-Peco Ultra.

DESTINATION

46

provide ideal conditions for ultra-running racing and training. During January, when the Big Bend Ultra is held, daytime temperatures are usually in the high sixties."

"Spending time in Big Bend is a powerful experience," Jamie Stone chimed in. "Just driving there is a massive undertaking, seven hours from Austin. The landscape wears away as you drive along I-10 and into the desert. It's vast, unforgiving and leaves you with a beautiful feeling of being alone. In the backcountry, it's so harsh that you are always analyzing your most fundamental needs and working to keep yourself centered and present in the moment, while at the same time fully aware of the enormity of the region and the geologic scale of our existence. Running in this region is like a spacewalk—you have to have all of your gear ready to go, and you have to execute a plan. For me, the beauty of the landscape is in the impression it leaves more than a series of clear, detailed moments."

The Big Bend Ultra began as a fifty-mile event and was originally held in Big Bend National Park, which adjoins Big Bend Ranch State Park to the east. It was first run in 2005. "We had roughly one hundred runners, and participants were very happy with the course," Carroll recalled. "However, the logistical challenges of the event—especially getting runners back to the starting point—were daunting." The race was moved to Big Bend Ranch the following year and continued to be fifty miles until 2017, when it was reimagined as a 50K (thirty-one-mile) event. The race begins and ends near Barton Warnock Visitor Center and rambles through the Fresno Creek drainage. Runners gradually gain one thousand feet of elevation on the way out and slowly lose that elevation on the way back. "Running the Fresno Creek drainage was deceivingly difficult," Jamie added. "Loose rocks, sand, pebbles, and harsh desert scrub dominate the course, making it difficult to get a firm footing and run at full speed. Sporadically the loose, dry arroyos turn into dense pockets of lush vegetation where the last drops of water are collected. It is a beautiful reminder of the significance of water. This race is a true test of mind and body."

If you've traveled far enough to compete in the Big Bend Ultra, you'll likely want to take some time to visit nearby Big Bend National Park. The Chisos Mountains dominate the northern side of the park, rising abruptly from the desert some five thousand feet. Thanks to their elevation, the Chisos attract a bit more moisture than the surrounding environs and support different flora than is found to the south, including aspen, Arizona cypress, ponderosa pine, and madrona. There are more than two hundred miles of established trails here. A few favorite hikes include Lost Mine, Window, and Mule Ears Spring. The Hot Springs Trail, six miles round-trip, takes you to—you guessed it—hot springs!

En route, take stock of the limestone path you're running on; in some spots, you may see ammonite fossils, which date back thirty-five million years. If you're seeking a more rigorous trail run, iRunFar.com recommends the South Rim Loop (14.5 or 17.5 miles, depending on your cutoff), which traverses the Chisos. A short distance into the run, you come to a significant climb that brings you into the mountains proper. When you reach the Southwest Rim near the middle of the loop, the mountains fall away dramatically.

Many visitors will carve out a day (or more) to see Big Bend's dramatic canyons—some 1,500 feet deep—from the Rio Grande. Tourists can enjoy day floats if the water is high enough, and a number of guide services have concessions to lead trips along the river.

P. CARROLL VOSS is a South Texas native, veteran endurance athlete, and fly-fishing enthusiast. He operates Overland Race Management (overlandracing.com), which provides course design, race directing, medical aid, HAM radio support, timing and results, and web production for trail-running and other endurance events.

JAMIE STONE is a Montessori teacher and runner based in Austin, Texas. He runs several marathons and ultras a year and can frequently be found exploring the labyrinth of trails in Austin's Greenbelt. You can keep up with his adventures on Instagram: @jstonejamie.

If You Go

▶ **Getting There:** The airport nearest to Big Bend is Midland/Odessa (250 miles from the Barton Warnock Visitor Center), which is served by United (800-864-8331; united.com) and American (800-433-7300; aa.com).
▶ **Best Time to Visit:** The Big Bend Ultra is held in mid-January. The park sees most of its visitors in the winter and early spring.
▶ **Race Information:** BigBend50.com highlights current race details and provides registration information.
▶ **Accommodations:** Both hotel rooms and campsites are available at Lajitas Golf Resort (432-424-5000; lajitasgolfresort.com). Visit Big Bend (visitbigbend.com) highlights other lodging options in the vicinity of the park.

DESTINATION

46

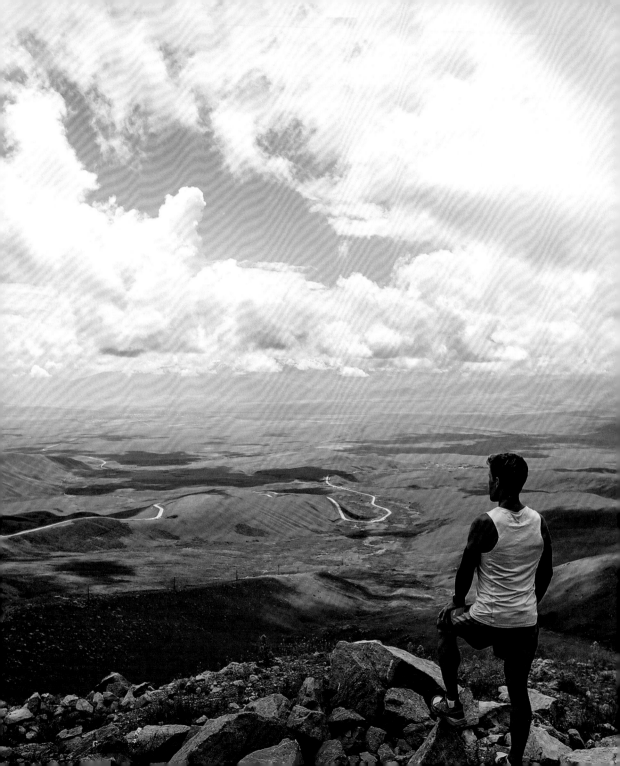

SILK ROAD

RECOMMENDED BY **Dean Karnazes**

Dean Karnazes has competed in organized road races. He has also run many adventure races off the beaten path. But until July of 2016, he had never run in the role of US diplomat.

"I was running in the San Francisco Marathon a few years back, and a guy came up and started chatting, as he recognized me," Dean began. "He'd read my book and said it kick-started his life. He explained that he worked for the State Department and was based in Kyrgyzstan . . . and that he wanted me to come and run in the footsteps of Alexander the Great, along the Silk Road. I thought he had a few loose marbles. But he followed up. What he had in mind was a bit of running-sports diplomacy. He brought in folks from the White House that were involved with the program. I realized it was legit—the roster of athletes included Cal Ripken, Shaquille O'Neal, and other notables. There had never been any runners. They wanted me to be the first.

"Their plan was for me to run through the 'Stans'—Uzbekistan, Kyrgyzstan, and Kazakhstan—tying together three different embassies because 2016 was going to be the twenty-fifth anniversary of these countries' independence from the Soviet Union. Something like this had never been done before. The idea was that sending in an ambassador who strips half-naked and runs down the middle of the street would create a positive impression. The power and commonality of running would unite people. It sounded great on paper, but when feet are on the street, running forty miles a day across the Stans can pose challenges. There's potential for things to go to hell in a handbasket fast." Overall, Dean would run 525 kilometers over eleven days.

For more than 1,500 years, the Silk Road connected East and West, fostering trade and laying the groundwork for the development of civilizations along its route, from China to

OPPOSITE:
Dean Karnazes
looks out over
Töö Ashuu
in the Kyrgyz
mountains,
more than
halfway through
his 525-kilometer
diplomacy
run along
the Silk Road.

DESTINATION

47

Rome. (The Silk Road was actually not one road, but a network of interconnected trade routes.) Uzbekistan, Kyrgyzstan, and Kazakhstan rest midway on the route, in the heart of central Asia. While no camels were involved, getting to Tashkent, Uzbekistan, was no easy task. "Coming from San Francisco, it was something like forty hours of travel time," Dean continued. "And twelve time zones. Coming off the plane, I was jet-lagged, sleep-deprived, it was 95 degrees . . . and hardly anyone spoke English. I was something like the tenth American to visit Uzbekistan in ten years. A State Department person drove me to my hotel and warned me that my room would be bugged. 'It's a throwback to the Soviet era,' he said. 'Look at how many smoke detectors there are.' That first day, I was whisked around the city and gave a speech at the embassy. The next day, I was running forty-two miles, crossing the border into Kyrgyzstan past guys with AK-47s. They stamped my passport, and I started running again."

Over the next ten days, Dean's schedule took on a similar tenor. "I'd run twenty or thirty miles across the desert or mountains and come into a township," he described. "The whole town would come out, as people had never seen an American. Bands would be playing, and a big spread of food would be presented. Though I was running and the food was heavy, I was advised that I had to try everything. Usually there was a big platter of horse meat—horse is a staple there—and a bowl of *kumis*, which is fermented mare's milk. I would equate it with drinking liquid Feta cheese. Then there would be a ceremony, a few photos, and then three or four more hours of running. Some people looked at me like I was a ghost—with my colorful running gear, Oakley sunglasses. I was certainly very different from anything they'd ever seen. But there is a commonality in running. My skin color was different, I didn't speak their language, I have a very different lifestyle, but when we run, we run the same way. When I passed, people would smile and wave, even if they had no idea of what I was doing. Sometimes kids would run alongside me . . . once they got over the shock of my appearance."

Dean was not alone in his travels. But his crew was somewhat different from those with whom he'd worked in the past. "I've done the Badwater® 135 before, and the crew I work with there is very smooth and efficient—like a military operation," Dean shared. "The van that accompanied me on my run had only one small door. There were eight people in the van. Every time it stopped, it was like a clown car . . . and they'd all get out and light up cigarettes. There was no cooler, just a bag with plastic bottles of water. I was dying from the heat and breathing in secondhand smoke. There were a few times along the way where we were supposed to stay with certain families, but they happened to not be home. But people were incredibly hospitable to take us into their yurts and feed us. Such hospitality is part of their nomadic culture."

Some of the terrain Dean crossed was quite arid and unfriendly to human endeavors, but there were nice surprises along the way as well. "The countryside of Kyrgyzstan was completely unspoiled," he described. "The rivers were filled with wild trout. That was one of my favorite meals—trout grilled over a flame with just a little salt. It was inspiring to see that there are places like this out there, so untouched in their natural state. I was also impressed by Almaty, the capital of Kazakhstan. It was very clean; the architecture and infrastructure were very modern. There's a ski resort like Squaw Valley just eight miles outside of town. I've seen many incredible cities, and Almaty was right up there."

Acting as an emissary of the United States, Dean met many influencers in central Asia. But his most memorable meeting may have been with a humble family. "It was my third day in Kyrgyzstan, and I was running into the mountains," he recalled. "A storm front came through, and it was hailing and raining. I was getting a little hypothermic. I passed a yurt and a family looked out. I smiled at them and they smiled back. The mother waved for me to come down, and she brought me into her home. She was cooking *kumis*, and the yurt was warm. I had some *kumis* and warmed up. We just smiled and pointed and laughed.

"I can't imagine what they thought. Here's this guy in funny clothes, running in the cold rain. But they were very welcoming and respectful."

DEAN KARNAZES has been hailed as one of the fittest men on the planet; *TIME* magazine named him one of the "Top 100 Most Influential People in the World." An internationally recognized endurance athlete and *New York Times* bestselling author, Dean has pushed his body and mind to inconceivable limits. Among his many accomplishments, he has run 350 continuous miles, foregoing sleep for three nights. He's run across Death Valley in 120-degree heat, and he's run a marathon to the South Pole at temperatures as low as –40 degrees. On ten different occasions, he's run a two-hundred-mile relay race solo, racing alongside teams of twelve. He also ran fifty marathons in fifty consecutive days, one in each US state, finishing with the New York City Marathon, which he ran in three hours flat. Dean and his incredible adventures have been featured on *60 Minutes*, *The Late Show with David Letterman*, *CBS News*, CNN, ESPN, *The Howard Stern Show*,

DESTINATION

47

NPR's *Morning Edition*, the BBC, and many others. He has appeared on the covers of *Runner's World* and *Outside* and has been featured in *Newsweek, People, GQ,* the *New York Times, USA TODAY,* the *Washington Post, Men's Journal, Forbes,* the *Chicago Tribune,* the *Los Angeles Times,* and the London *Telegraph.* He is a monthly columnist for *Men's Health,* the largest men's publication in the world. Learn more about Dean at ultramarathonman. com.

If You Go

▶ **Getting There:** Tashkent is served via Moscow by Aeroflot (888-340-6400; aeroflot.ru) and via Seoul by Korean Air (800-438-5000; koreanair.com).

▶ **Best Time to Visit:** Most visitors will travel to central Asia in the more clement months—between May and October.

▶ **Running Information:** Recreational running is not a highly developed activity in central Asia. You can learn more about Dean's travels at the Bureau of Educational and Cultural Affairs website (eca.state.gov/ultramarathon).

▶ **Accommodations:** The larger cities (like Tashkent and Almaty) have a smattering of western-style hotels. Along the rural sections of his route, Dean and his support crew would often arrange lodgings on the fly with local residents.

DESTINATION

47

KILLINGTON SPARTAN BEAST

RECOMMENDED BY **Jason Jaksetic**

The word "Spartan" implies both austerity and bravery. Jason Jaksetic found elements of each in a new kind of endurance race that was born in the Green Mountains of Vermont.

"In the 2000s, I was a hypercompetitive triathlete," he recalled. "I went to the Ironman Championships in Kona as an amateur, and it was my goal to eventually go professional. In 2009, I broke my hip before the Ironman Louisville. I went into a dark depression. A friend of mine was working for the Peace Corps in Swaziland (Africa), and I went to stay with him for two months. I went from a world where I wouldn't deign to ride anything less than a $10,000 bike to watching kids share a bike from 1975 to ride ten kilometers to school. I realized that I would need a change when I got back to America. I'd become a super-programmed 'wanker triathlete.' And triathlons had become, in some ways, a pampered thing; if I didn't get my GU [energy gel] at mile four, I'd fall apart!

"On the plane ride home, I lost my passport. A flight attendant gave me a passport that I thought was mine, but when I looked at it later I realized it belonged to a guy named Joe De Sena. I googled him and saw that he worked on Wall Street, lived in Vermont, and had done a number of crazy endurance events. When I returned his passport, I asked for a job. He said, 'I'm getting out of Wall Street, but I'm going to start a company in Vermont. Come up and join me.' I moved into his barn on an organic farm near Mount Killington. The company he was imagining would become Spartan. It was about back-to-basics endurance—pick up a big rock and walk up a mountain. No $10,000 bikes, no personal trainer plans. It channeled the idea that as humans, we are (or at least *were*) rugged animals. In 2011, this was a cultural shift. With Spartan, we were asking people to do some weird things. It was CrossFit meets *Jackass* [the MTV reality show featuring dangerous and ludicrous stunts] meets old-school fitness."

213

Killington sits toward the center of the Green Mountain State. Its namesake ski resort boasts the largest skiable area in the East. "The ski slopes of Killington were in use in the winter and could be ridden by mountain bikers in the summer," Jason continued. "When we started running up and down the trails, the mountain became a recreational playground for athletes who thought running up four miles could be fun, and it extended the season. Vermont is an experimental place, from a cultural perspective, going back to the hippies that came in the sixties and seventies and never left. That vibe has certainly benefited Spartan. I didn't feel out of place carrying a fifty-pound sandbag down Main Street. It's also helped that Vermont has open land laws, which protect landowners from being sued if someone gets injured on their land. You can sit down in a valley and pick a mountaintop and run up there, so long as the land isn't posted. You don't need to take a beaten path; you can choose your own. All these characteristics made Killington an ideal place for Spartan to develop the first Beast race."

Spartan races combine running with overcoming various obstacles (climbing over and under walls, carrying heavy objects, traversing monkey bars, etc.). They come in a variety of punishing flavors, including the Spartan Sprint (three-plus miles of obstacle racing, twenty-plus obstacles), the Spartan Super (eight-plus miles, twenty-five-plus obstacles), the Spartan Beast (thirteen-plus miles, thirty-plus obstacles), and the Spartan Ultra Beast (twenty-six-plus miles, sixty-plus obstacles). The events' "back to basics" ethos has struck a resonant chord—in 2017, there were more than two hundred Spartan events in more than thirty countries, and more than one million global participants. "Participating in a Spartan race is a tribal experience," Jason described. "All over the country there are people who don't quite fit in at their running club or gym. They come to our event, a muddy festival on the side of a mountain, and see thousands of other people who are into it. You feel at home, competing with people from many different walks of life who all see this as a fun activity. The human animal was made to run, jump, hang, and swing, and you'll do all that at a Spartan event. The races are timed, and they are competitive. But most athletes have the attitude that they're competing against last year's time."

The Spartan Beast at Killington is generally slated for the early fall to maximize the chances of having the race unfold against the blazing reds and oranges of foliage season. Jason likened the course to something from a J. R. R. Tolkien novel. "It's thirteen miles on the side of a mountain, on trails and in the woods, with monsters [in the shape of obstacles] positioned every half mile. It's about going on an adventure, not just covering thirteen miles. The climbs using vertical cargo nets are very uncomfortable for some; you're thirty feet up with only hay bales below. And there are the famously long barbed wire crawls, where you're in the mud."

Jason recalled a moment when the beautiful simplicity of the Spartan struck home. "I was participating in an Ultra Beast. You're allowed to drop a bag at the halfway point. I walked in cold, miserable, and exhausted and couldn't imagine going back out for the second half. I had stashed a dozen Buffalo wings in my bag, and covered in mud and cut up, I devoured them. As I ate them, I realized that this was an adventure—and I was like an animal running through the woods, trying not to die. There were no GU packets, no clocks. It was simple fun. I smiled, went outside, and kept motoring on."

JASON JAKSETIC is Spartan's go-to guy for all things training, fitness, and nutrition. He's completed double-Ironman distance triathlons and Spartan's grueling Ultra Beasts races. As one of the original modern-day Spartans, Jason helped develop the brand while living in the barn of Joe De Sena, Spartan's founder and CEO. He currently serves as Spartan's lifestyle editor and brand manager.

If You Go

▶ **Getting There:** Killington is roughly three hours from Boston and 1.5 hours from Burlington, Vermont, which are both served by most major domestic carriers.
▶ **Best Time to Visit:** The Killington Spartan Beast is generally run in late September or early October. The trails at Killington are free of snow for running from late May to early November.
▶ **Race Information:** Everything you need to know about the race in Killington—and other Spartan events—can be found at spartan.com.
▶ **Accommodations:** An extensive list of lodging options around Killington resides at killington.com.

DESTINATION

48

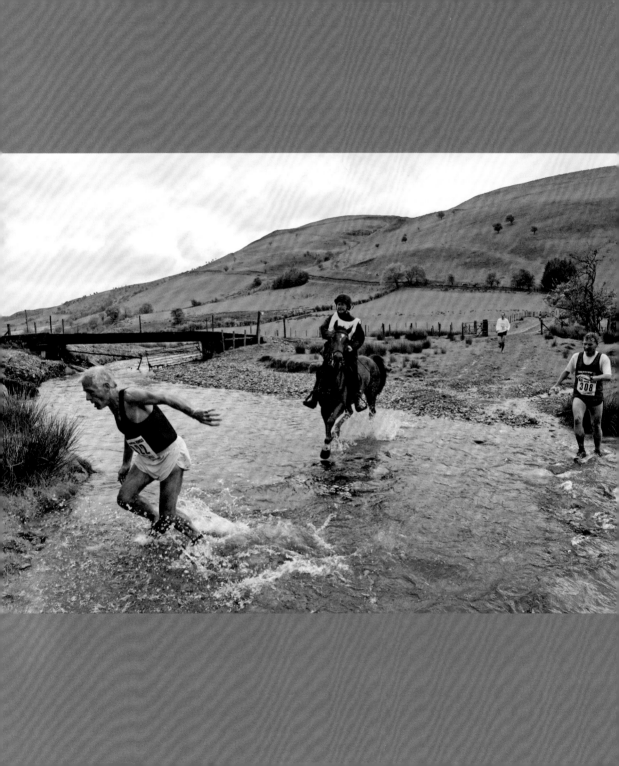

WHOLE EARTH MAN V. HORSE MARATHON

RECOMMENDED BY **Bob Greenough**

More often than not, the slightly mad notions that are spawned late in the evening at the local pub slowly disintegrate in the cool, cruel light of morning. But once in a great while, they can give birth to an event like the Whole Earth Man v. Horse Marathon, held each June in the Welsh town of Llanwrtyd Wells.

"Llanwrtyd Wells has been reliant on tourism for its economy for a long time," Bob Greenough began. "Mineral waters were discovered in 1732 and were found to be a cure for scurvy. By the Victorian era, Llanwrtyd Wells had become popular as a spa town. The spas also brought the railway to town; they supported a good number of small hotels and bed-and-breakfasts. In the 1930s and '40s, spa tourism fell off. The National Health Service had launched, and people no longer needed the waters to ease their aches and pains. Pony trekking was the next activity that brought visitors to town. At the time, many of the farms in the region were not mechanized, and the farmers were happy to rent their horses out. But soon diesel tractors arrived, and the pony trekking trade went away. By the 1970s, you had just a few walkers coming through, not enough to fill the many rooms here.

"In 1979, the landlord of one of the hotels (Neuadd Arms), Gordon Green, got into a discussion with a local huntsman at the hotel's back bar. Gordon, a runner, believed that a man could cover a certain distance quicker than a horse. The huntsman disagreed, and this was a topic of conversation each time the huntsman stopped by for a pint. Gordon saw an opportunity to promote Neuadd Arms and Llanwrtyd Wells, and eventually proposed the first Man v. Horse Marathon, which was run in 1980. I should say that the notion of a man outrunning a horse has some precedent in Welsh history. There was a fellow named Guto Nyth Bran who made a good few pounds betting horsemen that he could beat them in six- or twelve-mile races.

OPPOSITE:
Runners and equestrians cross several streams in the course of the Whole Earth Man v. Horse Marathon. Since the first running in 1980, human competitors have prevailed only twice.

DESTINATION

49

"That first year, only thirty or forty people showed up. But it was a curiosity, and the event grew a bit each year. Now we're up to roughly one thousand participants. That first year, the huntsman won the race, and the horse and rider would prevail the next twenty-three years. But the twenty-fifth year, the publican was proven right."

The Man v. Horse Marathon course showcases the beauty of the central Wales countryside, a region of low, rugged mountains, forests, and farmland. It should be noted that "marathon" is a bit of a misnomer. The length of the race has vacillated from nineteen to twenty-six miles since 1980. These days, the run is measured at twenty-two miles; human runners are given a fifteen-minute head start on the horses, and fifteen minutes are subtracted from the horses' times at the end. "Since the course goes through farm and forest areas, it changes with some regularity to accommodate the landowners," Bob continued. "Though it evolves, variations have been organic, and most agree it's a pig of a course—which is to say, challenging. There's very little flat land on this loop. If you're not going up or down a hill, you're standing still. You're running on a variety of surfaces—grass, rocky scree, thick mud, bogs, macadam—and there are several streams you need to cross. There are also some very narrow passages as you make your way down the mountains, ravines that you need to pick your way through. Horses don't do as well going downhill, or in narrow parts of the trail. Humans have an advantage on the steep downs. The most competitive runners know to let their legs go as fast as possible on these stretches."

At first blush, the idea of a man ever being able to outrun a horse seems slightly preposterous. Horses have four legs versus man's two; thoroughbreds can achieve speeds of more than forty miles per hour. But man does have certain tortoise-to-the-hare types of advantages. These include inner ears that help us stay balanced, springy tendons that make our strides efficient, and sweat glands that let us lose heat while we run. Research by Dan Lieberman, a professor of human evolutionary biology at Harvard, suggests that humans became good runners to become better hunters, pursuing animals persistently across the savanna until their prey succumbed to heat exhaustion.

It was in 2004 that man finally prevailed: Londoner Huw Lobb posted a time of two hours, five minutes, and nineteen seconds, besting his nearest equine opponent by two minutes. "A few years before, the bookmaker William Hill had pledged to pay one thousand pounds for each year that the race hadn't been won by a human," Bob added. "Huw pocketed twenty-five thousand." As of this writing, man has prevailed on only one other occasion.

The fact that runners have notched but two victories in nearly forty years of competition has done little to dampen the friendly, frolicking nature of the Man v. Horse Marathon. "We get a few elite athletes in to participate each year, but most take it quite casually," Bob described. "For a good number [of participants], I'd say it's the only competition they do each year, and 50 percent of our runners are only too keen to be done with the race and get to the pub. It's an event to take part in because your friends are doing it, rather than one that you strive to win, and you see people from all walks of life mingling together. For me, the best bit of the event is seeing the town on race day. Llanwrtyd Wells—the smallest town in the United Kingdom, by the way—has only six hundred residents; on an average day, you might see two or three people out and about. On race day, the town is overflowing, and everyone is smiling."

BOB GREENOUGH is part of the team at Green Events, the organizer of the Whole Earth Man v. Horse Marathon. He works primarily on this event, but also works on other events, including the World Mountain Bike Chariot Race Championships. Bob started racing in the mid-nineties, after years spent playing football, cricket, and golf. He regularly ran with his previous employer's running team in the annual World Airline Road Race in various places around the world, including San Francisco; Fort Worth, Texas; Kuala Lumpur; and Hamburg, Germany. Bob believes his greatest achievement has been raising five healthy, happy children with his wife.

If You Go

▶ **Getting There:** The Mid Wales region is within a two- to three-hour drive from airports in Cardiff, Liverpool, Manchester, and Birmingham, and a four-hour drive from London.
▶ **Best Time to Visit:** The Whole Earth Man v. Horse Marathon is held in early June.
▶ **Race Information:** Green Events (+44 01591610666; www.green-events.co.uk) manages the event. Interested participants can enter online.
▶ **Accommodations:** Visit Wales (visitwales.com) highlights lodging options and other attractions around Llanwrtyd Wells.

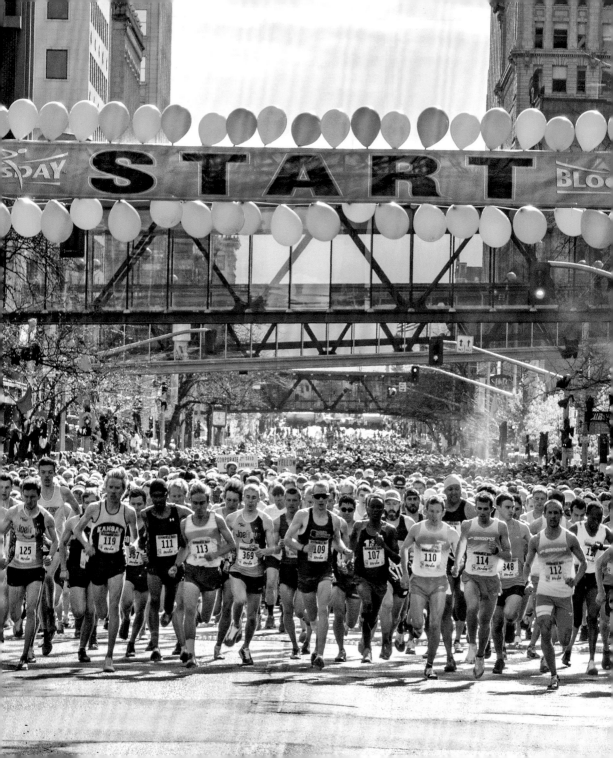

LILAC BLOOMSDAY RUN

RECOMMENDED BY **Don Kardong**

Don Kardong grew up in the wet (though not quite yet hip) Seattle area. But even in high school, he had his sights set on the drier side of the Evergreen State. "I started running as a sophomore in high school," he recalled. "Around that time, the best high school runner in the country was Gerry Lindgren, and he was from Spokane. I had a fascination with Gerry, and by extension, Spokane. It turned out that a track and field teammate of mine in college had grown up there. One summer he asked me if I had any interest in working at a summer camp in the region where he had a job. I went and decided that I liked the climate—warmer and drier than Seattle, especially in the summer. As an odd coincidence, it also turned out that the camp director had been Gerry's high school coach. When I finished college and had received my teaching certificate, I decided that I'd only apply for jobs in Spokane. I found one, teaching sixth grade.

"Before I arrived, I'd thought of Spokane as a big running town. But when I got there and would be out training, I didn't notice any other runners. I wondered, 'Where are they?' Right before the 1976 Olympics (in Montreal), I was invited to compete in the Peachtree Race in Atlanta, and I thought that having two thousand runners racing through downtown Atlanta was awesome—and that it was something Spokane could support. After the Olympics I pitched the idea to a reporter at the local paper (the *Spokesman-Review*), and that got the ball rolling. The mayor of Spokane at the time [David Rogers] had grown up in Boston and had fond memories of the Boston Marathon, so he thought it was a great thing. Spokane had hosted the World's Fair in 1974, and the downtown had been renovated for that event. The idea was that a downtown run would showcase what the city had become. We expected about three hundred runners to show up for the first Lilac Bloomsday Run, but we had 1,200. The original course took runners across

OPPOSITE:
The Lilac Bloomsday Run casts a spotlight on the city of Spokane in Washington's northeast corner.

221

DESTINATION

50

a toll bridge in town. That first year, I was in the lead when we crossed the bridge. I remember the toll takers with big smiles as I ran past, with Frank Shorter not far behind. [Frank would go on to win.] We didn't have to flip them a dime to pass. By the third year, there were so many people, the bridge was vibrating. People farther back in the pack could feel it undulating. There was also a big bottleneck getting onto the bridge. The next year, the toll bridge was no longer on the course."

Spokane frequently takes a backseat to Seattle as Washington cities go, yet it has much to recommend itself, especially for outdoors lovers. With a population of roughly two hundred thousand, Spokane is big enough to support a thriving food and cultural scene, but not so big as to make one feel anonymous. Many rivers (including the Spokane, which bifurcates the downtown) offer white-water rafting, kayaking, and fishing opportunities; nearby mountains offer ample snow sport and hiking options. "The thing I learned about Spokane is that the city doesn't overwhelm the surrounding area," Don continued. "It's easy to get outside the city to some great running areas. There's one state park three miles from downtown where you can run forever." Like many other western cities, Spokane has attracted many who enjoy fitness and the outdoors. That helps explain how this 12K in a relatively remote and sparsely populated region has attracted as many as sixty thousand entrants . . . though runners come from far and wide to participate. "If you talk to people who are part of a running group anywhere in the country, chances are good they've heard of Bloomsday," Don added.

The twelve-kilometer course showcases both downtown Spokane and the Spokane River Gorge, which runners cross several times. "There's a good bit of up and down on the route," Don explained, "as you're dropping into the gorge and then climbing out. There are also three big hills. The third of the hills—Doomsday—is the biggest challenge, at least in part because you can see the whole hill in front of you as you approach. At the top of Doomsday Hill, there's a guy who dresses up as a vulture. He's been doing this for almost thirty years. Lots of runners like to stop for a selfie with the vulture. Given the difficulty of the course, I'm constantly amazed at some of the fast times that are posted." The field at Bloomsday any given year will have its share of youth runners thanks to "Fit for Bloomsday . . . Fit for Life," a training program that introduces elementary school children to running. "We've had almost eight thousand kids sign up for the 2017 program," Don said. "The younger kids might not do the run, but many of the fourth and fifth graders do. Race finishers get a T-shirt only after they've finished, and you can be pretty sure that the kids who finish the race wear their T-shirts—which feature a special design that's only revealed the day of the race—to school the next day."

The T-shirts are a point of pride among Bloomsday finishers. Don recalled how one participant responded to his T-shirt. "One year, I happened to be watching the TV coverage of the race. The crew was there at the finish line to interview some of the first runners to cross—often, runners from Kenya. One of the Kenyan participants had picked up his shirt, which that year was bright blue. The reporter asked him what he thought of the shirt, and the runner replied, 'I think it's beautiful, and I'll take it back to my home in Kenya and put it on the wall so I can always remember running in Bloomsday.'

"Someday, I hope to visit Kenya and see that shirt on the wall of his home."

DON KARDONG grew up in the Seattle area, graduated from Stanford University in 1971, received a second bachelor's degree and a teaching certificate from the University of Washington in 1974, and moved to Spokane that year to take a job as an elementary school teacher. In 1976, Don finished fourth in the marathon at the Olympics in Montreal, and the next spring he founded the Lilac Bloomsday Run. In 1977 he left teaching to open a retail sporting goods store in downtown Spokane, and after selling the business in 1986 he pursued a career as a writer, primarily for *Runner's World* magazine, for the next sixteen years. From 2002 to 2004 Don served as executive director of the Mobius Children's Museum in Spokane. In August of 2004, after many years as a member of Bloomsday's board of directors, he took over as race director. Don is married and has two grown daughters.

If You Go

▶ **Getting There:** Spokane is served by several carriers, including Alaska Airlines (800-252-7522; alaskaair.com) and United (800-864-8331; united.com).

▶ **Best Time to Visit:** The Lilac Bloomsday Run is held on the first Sunday in May.

▶ **Race Information:** Everything you need to know resides at bloomsdayrun.org.

▶ **Accommodations:** Visit Spokane (888-SPOKANE; visitspokane.com) highlights a host of lodging options in the city and surrounding region.

DESTINATION

50

Library of Congress Control Number: 2017949400

ISBN: 978-1-4197-2912-6
eISBN: 978-1-68335-238-9

Text copyright © 2018 Chris Santella

Photography credits: Page 2: © Drew Levin for NYRR; Pages 8, 208: © U.S. Department of State;
Page 12: © Modfos/Shutterstock.com; Pages 14, 98: © UTMB® Archives – Franck Oddoux; Page 16:
© Tyler Deniston; Pages 20, 76, 134, 142: © Marathon Tours; Pages 25, 170: © Myke Hermsmeyer; Page 28:
© Super Sport Images; Page 32: © Courtesy of The Vancouver Sun, a division of Postmedia Network Inc; Page
36: © Scott Walmsley/Shutterstock.com; Page 42: © Chris Kostman/Badwater 135; Page 46: © Yoon Kim; Page
50: © Bob Cullinan Photo; Page 54: © Bay to Breakers; Page 58: © Keith Facchino; Page 64: © Conquer the Wall
Marathon; Page 68: © BolderBOULDER; Page 72: © Reid Delman; Page 82: © Rena Schild/Shutterstock.com;
Page 86: © Bikeworldtravel/Shutterstock.com; Page 90: © Dan Vernon/Great Run; Page 102: © Sergieiev/
Shutterstock.com; Page 106: © Atlanta Track Club/Paul Kim; Page 110: © mkrberlin/Shutterstock.com; Page 114:
© Anastasios71/Shutterstock.com; Page 118: © Hawaii Marathon; Page 122: © Bank of America Chicago Marathon;
Page 126: © Iryna Dzvonkovska/Shutterstock.com; Page 130: © Karen Fuchs – Reggae Marathon; Page 138:
© Eston Photography by Mike Trummel for the Crescent City Classic; Page 146: © Dave Dostie; Page 150:
© Ben Kimball; Page 154: © Fay Foto/Boston; Page 158: © Craig Zabransky; Page 162: © Kathleen Swinehart;
Page 166: © Grandma's Marathon; Page 174: © Joe Tabacca/Shutterstock.com; Page 178: © Naruedom
Yaempongsa/Shutterstock.com; Page 184: © Todd Bosworth; Page 188: © Kayla Young; Page 192: © Andes
Adventures; Page 196: © Albatross Adventure Marathons; Page 200: © Chattanooga Times Free Press Photo;
Page 204: © Aaron Bates; Page 216: © Alamay; Page 220: © Tom Duncan

Jacket © 2018 Abrams

Editor: Ashley Albert
Designer: Anna Christian
Production Manager: Kathleen Gaffney

This book was composed in Interstate, Scala, and Village.

Printed and bound in China
10 9 8 7 6 5 4 3 2 1

Abrams Image books are available at special discounts when purchased in quantity for premiums and
promotions as well as fund-raising or educational use. Special editions can also be created to specification.
For details, contact specialsales@abramsbooks.com or the address below.

ABRAMS The Art of Books
195 Broadway, New York, NY 10007
abramsbooks.com